REHEALTH YOURSELF

Eat Great, Lose Weight and Improve Your Total
Health Now!

Chef John Shirk
www.rehealthyourself.com

Notice

This book is intended as a reference, not as a medical manual. The information given is to help you make better decisions about your health. It is not intended as a substitute for any treatment that may have been prescribed by your doctor. If you suspect you have a medical condition, you are urged to see a doctor before starting anything in this book.

Dedication

I was inspired by my father to write this cookbook who at 38 years old had to start watching what he ate due to heart disease. My mother who is an excellent cook has continuously studied food and how simple changes can affect your health. They have encouraged me to get the word out and have taught me much more than they realize. Thank you so much for your continued support! I Love You!

REHEALTH YOURSELF

Eat Great, Lose Weight and Improve Your Total Health Now!

Chef John Shirk
www.rehealthyourself.com

Contents

Foreword

As a personal trainer, I know that food and nutrition are closely related, but are not the same thing. Food is anything that we eat, but nutrition is necessary to live. For many years, we have been eating to suppress hunger, but not necessarily to satisfy our bodies' needs. As a result, our bodies are suffering. According to the Centers for Disease Control, the top two causes for chronic disease are poor nutrition and lack of exercise. Our bodies have not changed much at all since paleolithic times, but our food on the other hand has changed drastically.

Modern food has been genetically modified, flavor-enhanced, and powerfully over-processed. Our soils have been depleted of nutrients by over fertilizing and over farming. However, most of our weight problems are even simpler than that. We simply do not eat real food. John's recipes in this book are designed to provide you with the nutrients, fiber, protein, and blood-sugar balancing foods that you need to get healthy, find your natural weight and maintain it.

I know only a handful of people who are completely happy with their weight. On the other hand, everyone else I know wishes they could lose x number of pounds. That's a huge majority. The most frustrating part for me as a personal trainer is that the majority want to lose weight overnight with a magic pill. They want to lose weight yesterday. They have no patience. Unfortunately, there is no magic pill for rapid weight loss. Losing weight takes patience if you want to do it right, keep it off, and be healthy.

Preparing real food does require more time than unwrapping a frozen dinner or opening a carry-out bag, but none of these recipes will require you to quit your job or give up your favorite TV show, and they taste better than any convenience option. It might even take you 30 minutes to prepare a meal, but that's ok! Give yourself permission to cook real meals at home in your kitchen and reap the health benefits that come with eating nutritious, delicious food.

Go ahead. Release your inner chef, and let Chef John lead you on your way to getting healthy again!

Julia Shirk Hughes, FNT
Founder, SmarterCity, LLC

Chapter 1

Introduction

Have you been to the doctor recently and were told you needed to lose weight? Maybe you were told your cholesterol was too high? Did the doctor tell you that if you do not make some changes soon, you may get diabetes? Have you felt sluggish and tired lately? Do you think you are overweight?

You know you need to make a change. *How am I going to do this?* You ask yourself. *Do I need a diet? What diet should I use?* You search for weight loss on the internet, only to discover there are thousands of diets. You then go to the library and, wow, hundreds of books. You are now very confused and feel helpless. There is so much information available that it can be very daunting, scary, and overwhelming. Which one will work for you?

Here is the good news: By picking up the *Rehealth Yourself* cookbook, you have taken the first step to changing your health. First of all, this cookbook is not a diet! Do not think or use the word "diet" any longer. A diet is something you start and stop. This cookbook will show you how to make a few simple changes, and by simply eliminating some foods and adding some others, you will improve your health. You will eat incredible, high-quality, natural food. You will add a little bit of exercise into your daily routine, and you will burn the excess fat in your body and get back to your natural healthy weight. These simple changes may also lower your blood sugar, improve your blood pressure, lower your "bad" cholesterol (LDL), raise your good cholesterol (HDL), and give you more energy. Yes, it really is that simple.

My Wake-Up Call

As a chef, I have spent many years thinking about writing a cookbook featuring healthy, delicious, and natural ingredients. My busy lifestyle caused me to put off my dream time and again. Then life provided me with a wake-up call: I recently realized I was overweight. The revelation came when I was looking at some photos after a spring fishing trip with my dad and brother. I saw a photo of myself and thought, "How did that bowling ball get in my gut?" I have always been a slim, athletic person. My height is 5'9 and my weight has typically ranged from 155-160 pounds for most of my adult life.

The day I saw the bowling ball in my gut, I weighed myself. To my surprise, the scale read 193 pounds. I WAS SHOCKED AND VERY CONCERNED! Then I realized that for the last year, I had been eating poorly. I found myself eating a lot of fast food. I would grab a sandwich or a quick junior burger at the drive-thru, thinking that just one would be okay. The problem was, pretty soon I was eating three or four sandwiches or junior burgers a week. Sometimes, if I was really hungry, I would order two at a time. I knew they weren't healthy, but being pressed for time, stressed out, and increasingly addicted to their high sodium and fat content, it was so easy to make excuses and gobble them down.

After seeing my new, unhealthy weight, I knew I needed to change. More than anything, I knew that being overweight was increasing my risk for heart disease. When I was a kid, my dad had severe heart problems, and I didn't want to develop them, too. I knew that the time had come to start writing this book and practicing what I preach.

My Family History of Heart Disease

It was 1974 and I was 10 years old, excited to be going to Camp Kern where my dad and I would join other campers with "The Indian Guides" for this annual event. The camp offered amazing activities that included hiking in the woods, crossing rivers and streams, climbing huge trees and boulders, and looking out over the vast valleys. It was on one of those hiking trips that I noticed my dad hiking more and more slowly. When we were about a mile away from camp, he said he wasn't feeling well and told one of the other fathers. I overheard my dad say he was having chest pains. Was he having a heart attack? How were we going to get him back? What were we going to do? I was scared. We started back to camp slowly, and after several stops, my dad returned safely.

We left for home that night, and the next morning my dad saw his doctor. The doctor scheduled several tests and two months later my dad underwent coronary bypass surgery. He was only 38 years old.

At that time, the go-to diet for those with heart disease was from The American Heart Association, who recommended foods that were "fat-free" or "low-fat." They recommended margarine instead of butter, and my dad was not allowed to eat eggs, nuts, olives and especially coconut, because they were too high in saturated fats. The 1974 version of a heart-healthy diet unfortunately resulted in people eating a lot of carbohydrates. My mom, being a very good cook, took these recommendations very seriously and ensured that my dad followed the diet.

Still, less than 8 years later, my dad's arteries were clogged again, and he underwent another 4 bypasses. The recommended diet at the time was still the same fat-free and low-fat eating plan that was considered beneficial. But just 5 years later, my dad needed to unclog his arteries again. He had his first heart attack and needed a procedure called an angioplasty. Dad was fixed up again, sent home, and told to keep eating so-called "healthy" foods. In January of 1995, my dad needed another bypass surgery. This would be his last one, as the doctor informed our family that they could do no more bypasses and recommended he see a specialist who treated high cholesterol and look into a new "Mediterranean diet."

The Mediterranean diet was discovered in 1950, and yet most doctors did not start to recommend it until the 1990s. My mom quickly researched the diet and made some changes to my dad's diet plan to reflect the new recommendations.

The diet recommended eating all natural foods, including those with good fats, such as nuts, seeds, lean meats, olive oil, and less processed carbohydrates. At this time, the doctor informed my brother and I that we were also at a greater risk for heart disease and that we needed to take care of ourselves. I never forgot that.

My Mission

Since becoming a chef, I have always tried to find the best healthy ingredients for my recipes. I do it for both my family and restaurant clientele. I believe that people want to eat the best food possible but do not always know what is in the food they consume.

For the last several years, I had worked as a Corporate Chef for one of the nation's largest food distributors. It was my job to test new products that large food companies wanted to sell. The first thing I would do when I received a new product was to read the label to see the ingredients, and I would almost always find myself asking questions: *Why are there preservatives in this? Is it necessary to add*

BHA or BHT? What is disodium inosinate? Are there food dyes? Added fats pumped into the food?

The answers I received usually included some variation of "These additives enhance the food, making it tastier/more tender/juicier." I was often told, "This is what the consumer wants to eat." What?!? Is this really what consumers want to eat? This food is being sold to restaurants and then sold to consumers as "fresh and natural". Consumers think they can feel good about these selections, but they don't know what's really in the food they are ordering and consuming.

You may be wondering how all of this is related to heart health and weight loss. With all of these additives, preservatives, higher sodium ingredients, sugars, and fats, what started out as natural food becomes processed food. It is nearly impossible to stay healthy and lose weight when your body is full of these processed foods and toxins. Actually, you are guaranteed to gain weight and become unhealthy.

The *Rehealth Yourself* cookbook is designed to restore your body to its prime condition and help you lose excess fat and weight the natural way. This is not a miracle lose-weight-fast program. Most of those programs only work for a short period of time. The *Rehealth Yourself* cookbook is a common sense guide to healthy eating. If you are overweight and follow the *Rehealth Yourself* cookbook carefully, you should expect to lose 2-4 pounds per week. Some people have lost over 6 pounds after the first week. You may also see improved cholesterol numbers, but most importantly higher HDLs and lower LDLs and triglycerides. Other potential benefits include lower blood sugar and lower blood pressure.

Only 10 weeks after discovering my bowling ball belly, my weight was down to 155 pounds—a whopping 38 pounds lighter! To put that in perspective, it's the weight equivalent of over three real bowling balls. I feel great. I have much more energy. I have been sleeping more soundly, and food now tastes even better than ever. Those junior burgers are a thing of the past, and to be honest, I don't miss them!

I often wonder what my weight and cholesterol numbers would have been if I had chosen quarter pounders instead of junior burgers or added french fries and a large soda to my order. I don't want to follow my dad into the operating room, and with my new plan, I'm doing everything I can to make sure that doesn't happen. The *Rehealth Yourself* cookbook will help you feel better than you have in years.

So let's get started!

Chapter 2

Your First Steps:
Small Steps That Will Change Your Life!

"The first and best victory is to conquer self."

Plato

1. See your doctor!

First and foremost, if you have not seen your doctor recently, schedule an appointment for a complete physical and ask for a complete cholesterol blood test. Tell your doctor that you want to start exercising and eating healthy, and after getting the "OK," tell him or her that by the next appointment, you will be a new, healthy person.

2. Start a journal.

- Write down your starting weight and your waist measurement or belt size.
- Buy a good quality scale. You should weigh yourself a few times per week.
- Record your cholesterol levels, blood pressure, and blood sugar numbers.
- Include in your journal this statement: **I AM NOT ON A DIET!** Tell yourself every day that you are not on a diet. A diet is something you start and stop if and when you reach your goal. The *Rehealth Yourself* cookbook is designed to

encourage a lifestyle change, not a diet. You are simply changing your eating habits and the food you consume.

3. If you smoke, quit!

I can list a thousand reasons why you should quit smoking. You probably already know most of them. Do it for yourself and your family. You have more help around you than ever before, so if one way doesn't work, try another. The benefits are instant and too great to ignore. For more information, go to www.helpguide.org [1] and search "smoking."

4. Try to get 7-8 hours of sleep.

Numerous studies have shown that not getting enough sleep increases your desire for sugar and carbohydrates. When you're tired, it's easy to just grab any kind of food. Poor sleep makes your brain tired and you do not think clearly, which can lead to unhealthy eating. Focus on getting a good night's sleep, and you will make better decisions and have more energy. For more information, check out www.bettersleep.org [2].

5. Control alcohol consumption.

A glass of red wine with a meal, a cold beer, or a vodka, soda, and lime with some friends are some of the pleasures of life. But drinking daily is a bad habit. Too much alcohol can do more harm than you realize, especially if you are overweight. Think about this: If you drink just 2 adult beverages per day, you will consume over 70,000 extra calories per year, which is equivalent to over 20 pounds of weight gain, mostly right in your belly. If you drink every day, try to stop for a month; this will help you lose weight much more quickly. Studies have shown that an occasional glass of red wine or a cocktail can actually be beneficial for heart health. An occasional adult beverage means 3-4 drinks per week. And remember, a drink equals 12 ounces of beer, 5 ounces of wine, or 1.5 ounces of liquor. For more information, visit www.cdc.gov/alcohol [3].

6. Reduce and manage stress.

Stress sets off a chain of events. First, you have a stressful situation that's usually upsetting but not harmful. Your body reacts by releasing the hormone adrenaline, that temporarily causes your breathing and heart rate to speed up and your blood pressure to rise. These reactions prepare you to deal with the situation by confronting it or by running away from it—the "fight or flight" response. When stress is constant, your body remains in high gear off and on for days or weeks at a time. The link between chronic or extreme stress and heart disease is not clear, but studies have shown that constant stress raises blood pressure, which can lead to heart disease and stroke. Other studies have shown that stressed out people tend to eat recklessly. For more information on dealing with stress, visit www.mayoclinic.org [4] and search "stress management."

7. Start to exercise.

WARNING!
If you are overweight, have any pre-existing medical conditions, or have not exercised recently, consult your doctor before beginning any exercise routine!

Aside from changing your diet, exercise is probably the single best medication for your overall health. Exercise speeds up your metabolism and burns calories and fat, improves your mood and reduces stress, boosts energy, and promotes better sleep. Make it a part of your daily life. When my father was diagnosed with heart disease, he was told to exercise regularly. From that day forward, he made a commitment. He started walking every day, starting with just a hundred yards, then going a quarter mile, and gradually increasing to 3 miles, or about 30-40 minutes at a time. Today, he has been walking for nearly 40 years. If he can't go outside, he walks on the treadmill, and when not walking, he keeps active by working in the garden, trimming bushes, or building things. My dad exercises for his heart, but it has also helped him maintain his optimal natural weight without fad diets.

Exercise can mean many different things, including taking a brisk walk for 30 minutes, practicing yoga for an hour, using an elliptical or treadmill, riding a stationary bike, walking the mall, using the track or bleacher steps at your local high school stadium, hiking, biking, or swimming. You do not have to do the same exercise over and over or even join a gym. Make it fun and be creative, or invite a friend to join you. You can even watch television while exercising. There are several exercise programs on TV—pick one and join in. Or, if your children have a gaming console like a Wii or an Xbox, play one of the numerous exercise and sports games they offer. Get your family involved, and all of a sudden, you will have put in a great workout!

Set your smart phone or calendar as a daily reminder to exercise. Some days will be tough, but if you just keep going, you will reap the rewards and improve your health naturally. After a short while, you will want to exercise! Remember your goal is to exercise 30 minutes per day, 6 days per week.

If you become really thirsty during exercise, this is a sign that you are dehydrated and need to consume more water a few hours prior to exercising.

8. Clean out your kitchen.

You will need to remove processed and unhealthy foods from your kitchen. Most of these foods have a long list of ingredients that include preservatives, high fat, and sugar. If you do not remove these items, it will be very tempting to keep grabbing little bites here and there. Here is a list of foods to remove:

Baked goods	Breadcrumbs
Baked beans	Breads
Chips	Cereals
Frozen entrees	Juices
Milk	Dressings
Snack bars	Candy
Soda/pop	Fruit-flavored yogurts
Crackers	Multi-grain anything

Anything with artificial sweeteners and/or HFCS (high fructose corn syrup)

This list could go on and on, but I think you get the idea. In Chapter 3, I will go into greater detail about the good foods you should eat and the bad foods you shouldn't eat.

9. Reconnect with your kitchen.

Listed below are a few pieces of equipment that will make food preparation and cooking in your kitchen much easier. I highly recommend the following:

- **A good-quality blender.** There are several blenders available, but my favorites are the Vitamix and Blendtech. Both are super powerful and reliable, but a little costly at $300-$500. If you do not want to spend that much, I also like the KitchenAid Diamond series. Although not as powerful, it will do the job at about a fourth of the price.

- **A handheld immersion blender.** I love the Cuisinart, which is very powerful and inexpensive. I use it almost every day.

- **A small food processor.** There are several on the market that are very good. You do not need a big one or one that offers over 100 pieces—just something small and simple.

- **A food thermometer.** There are several different kinds, from digital to no-frills. Just make sure the temperature range is between 32 degrees and 175 degrees.

- **A set of good-quality chef knives and a knife sharpener.** This is very important because you will be using knives frequently to cut and prepare food. A knife sharpener is essential for keeping your quality knives sharp, which makes food preparation much easier and safer.

Here are a few more helpful items for your kitchen:
- Non-slip cutting boards
- Measuring cups and utensils (plastic or stainless steel)
- Small, medium, and large whisks (stainless steel and silicon)
- Small and large high-heat rubber spatulas

Physical #1

Three months after starting the *Rehealth Yourself* lifestyle:

I arrived at the doctor's office for my annual physical, having fasted for the recommended 12 hours so I could have my blood drawn for the cholesterol test. The nurse first checked my weight, and when she entered my weight into the computer system, a warning appeared. She asked if I felt okay, and I said I had never felt better. She asked if I was aware that I had lost more than 10 percent of my weight since my last physical. I replied yes, I actually had lost closer to 20 percent and that I had changed my diet. The nurse also checked my blood pressure and stated that it was excellent.

During my physical, the doctor was very pleased to find out that I had lost weight by eating healthy and exercising. He was very interested to see the lab reports for my cholesterol test. I left the doctor and headed down to the first floor to have my blood drawn. Later that day, I received an email from my doctor:

"In comparison to your last lipid profile (one year earlier), your HDL has improved, your LDL, VLDL and triglycerides have all decreased. You're doing a great job overall. I have no other special recommendations for any changes.
I will see you at your next visit. Please be sure to adhere to the diet and exercise regime that you described in the office."

After reading the email, I sat back for a minute and thought, *Wow, I have only changed my diet and lifestyle for 3 months, and I have achieved these results. Is it really that simple to Rehealth Yourself?*

Chapter 3

DITCH IT:
Foods Not to Consume

"You must do the things you think you cannot do."

Eleanor Roosevelt

In this chapter, you will learn what foods cause havoc in your body so you can eliminate them from your diet. Earlier I listed what foods you should remove from your kitchen, and at first, this may seem like a major task and may even be difficult. But stick with it, and in a very short period of time, it will become easy and feel natural to you.

To begin, you will need to eliminate white or processed foods from your diet. White foods have "bad carbs," which are less satisfying than "good carbs."[5] The body absorbs processed grains and simple sugars relatively quickly. This creates an increase in blood sugar and triggers a release of insulin, and an hour or two after eating, hunger returns.

White foods include refined flours like all-purpose flour. White processed flour has a very high glycemic rate that quickly raises the blood sugar level and insulin levels, which can be a direct cause of diabetes. As Mark Hyman, MD, [6] explains, "The biggest problem is processed wheat, the major source of gluten in our diet. The history of wheat parallels the history of chronic disease and obesity across the world. It is not just the amount but also the hidden components of wheat that drive weight gain and disease. This is not the wheat your great-grandmother used to bake her bread. It is FrankenWheat—a scientifically engineered food product developed in the last 50 years." Due to the inflammation properties of wheat, you will also want to stay away from products labeled "wheat," "whole wheat," "100% wheat" and "multi-grain" for now as they do not help with weight loss. Eliminate wheat for now and you will quickly see the benefits. Once you reach your optimal health, you can try wheat again if you want. You may not want to after you've seen the results! As a chef, I love bread, so I occasionally have a piece of sprouted wheat toast. I do notice that if I eat wheat for 2 days in a row, my belt size will get tighter. I have done this test over and over. After you have lost your excess weight, try it for yourself.

Examples of white foods to avoid are bagels, breads, cakes, crackers, cookies, danishes, ice cream, potato chips, pasta, pretzels, white rice, and sugar-sweetened drinks.

You must eliminate these foods to kick start your weight loss and get your health heading in the right direction.

Another white food that you must ditch is "added sugar." Natural sugar in whole foods like fruits, vegetables, beans, and grains is good sugar. When simple sugars are naturally found in whole food, they come with vitamins, minerals, protein, and fiber. The presence of fiber makes a big difference because it slows down the absorption of sugar and moderates its impact on blood sugar. When any type of sugar is added to foods during processing, however, you consume calories without the nutrients or fiber. This kind of sugar is bad sugar. Your body is probably addicted to sugar, since it is found in many processed foods and drinks. Once the unhealthy refined sugars are removed from your body, I promise that you will start to feel better. It will also help make it easier for you to eliminate other white foods.

I also recommend ditching "fake sugars," otherwise known as artificial sweeteners such as aspartame, saccharin, and sucralose. These products may be low in calories, but they stimulate the brain into wanting more sweets. There is some evidence to suggest that these products may cause some serious side effects such as headaches, migraines, irritable bowel syndrome, and even cancer. These sweeteners can be found in just about everything from diet soda, chewing gum, frozen desserts and cough syrup, so reading labels is a must!

In a short period of time you will no longer miss sugar. While there are many types of natural sugars on the market, most are still not recommended. When I developed my "bowling ball belly," I was using 1-2 teaspoons of organic raw sugar per cup of coffee, and drinking 2-3 cups per day. I would sometimes also have a few iced teas. I was consuming a lot of sugar every day, but I didn't notice. Small amounts can add up to large amounts very easily.

When I made the decision to get rid of the bowling ball, I switched to organic raw coconut crystals and dropped my serving size down to ⅛ of a teaspoon. I realized that reaching for a teaspoon and adding sugar was a habit that I had built over time. It took just a few days to adjust. Now, I don't use any sweeteners in my beverages, and I don't miss them.

Sugar hides under many names. Here is a list of some added sugars to avoid: brown sugar, cane crystals, cane sugar, corn sweetener, corn syrup, crystalline fructose, dextrose, evaporated cane juice, fructose, fruit juice concentrates, glucose, high fructose corn syrup, lactose, malt syrup, maltodextrin, maltose, rice syrup, sucrose, and xylose. There are many other disguises for sugar as well, so if you do not know what an ingredient is, search for it on the internet.

In addition to white foods, you should also avoid fruit juices. These beverages have a ton of added sugar, are made from concentrate, or naturally contain high amounts of sugar. Instead of ingesting all that sugar, replace your beverages with filtered ice water, green tea, or some morning 50/50 coffee (half decaf/half regular). Seltzer water and coconut water are also great choices and available in many flavors. Make sure there are no added sugars, additives, or preservatives.

Sometimes, I hear people say, "But I can't drink water!" WHAT? That's like saying you can't breathe oxygen. Of course you can drink water! Your body contains 55-65% water. You *need* water because you are human. Whenever I ask why someone can't drink water, I hear, "I just can't drink it." The real problem is that these people have probably forgotten what real water tastes like, because it's not loaded with artificial flavors and sweetened. Well, you picked up this book for a reason, and water will help you get healthy. It's basically free and tastes great, not to mention it keeps you hydrated and feeling full. So what's the problem? Get drinking!

Chapter 4

SUPER FOODS FOR SUPER HEALTH

"You may delay, but time will not."
Benjamin Franklin

In this chapter, I share with you my favorite super foods that will help improve your health. Super foods are full of natural antioxidants and nutrients. The super foods listed below have been tried and tested and are known for their health and weight loss properties. This list isn't exhaustive; the foods mentioned here are just my favorites, but there are many great foods with high antioxidants and nutrients that are excellent for both health and weight loss. Don't be afraid to try something new. If you don't like one super food, just try another. I'm positive that you will find many to fall in love with.

Chef John's Recommended Super Foods

Nuts

As a natural whole food, nuts are excellent sources of antioxidants, vitamins, and minerals that can boost your health in numerous ways above and beyond weight control. In a new review of 31 trials [7], people who ate extra nuts or substituted nuts for other foods lost about 1.4 extra pounds and half an inch from their waistlines.

Almonds

My favorite nuts are almonds. Almonds are a great super food because they are rich in healthy fats that will help you lose weight. Just by eating a few almonds instead of crackers, chips, or cookies, you will be giving yourself natural fiber and protein, ingredients that are great weight loss promoters. You will feel full much longer and have some extra energy as well.

Almonds are high in calories and fat, but the fat is monounsaturated, otherwise known as "the good fat." These fats are healthy for your heart and give your metabolism a boost to burn off the excess "bad" fat. When purchasing almonds, I recommend only buying raw, skin-on, unsalted almonds.

Walnuts

Just like almonds, walnuts are high in good fats, fiber, and protein. They also help lower LDL cholesterol (the "bad" guy) and provide benefits to the heart. I like to mix walnuts and almonds together. Just like almonds, I recommend you only buy your walnuts raw and unsalted.

One small word of caution when it comes to nuts: The benefits of nuts are great, but it can be easy to overeat them. Your daily intake shouldn't exceed 1-2 ounces or ¼ cup of nuts daily, which is about as much as you can hold in the palm of your hand.

Seeds

Chia Seeds

Chia seeds were revered by the ancient Aztec and Mayan empires as vital nourishment. These mighty seeds are packed with omega-3 fatty acids, protein, rare antioxidants, and fiber. Only 1 tablespoon of chia seeds provides 20% of your recommended daily fiber intake, as well as 3 grams of protein. Their mild, nutty flavor makes them easy to add to foods and beverages. They are great to blend into healthy shakes and can also be sprinkled on vegetables. Learn to love the chia seed!

Flax Seeds

Flax seeds are one of nature's richest plant sources of omega-3 fatty acids. These fatty acids are "essential" fats the human body needs for many functions, from building healthy cells to maintaining brain and nerve function. Our bodies can't produce them, so we need them from food. One serving of flax seeds contains almost 20% of your daily recommended natural fiber, a sure way to help with weight loss.

Pumpkin Seeds

Pumpkin seeds are one of nature's almost perfect foods. A natural source of amino acids and unsaturated fatty acids, they contain most B vitamins, along with C, D, E, and K. Pumpkin seeds are high in protein, at 9.75 grams per ¼ cup. I like to mix pumpkin seeds with almonds and walnuts for a healthy energy boost and filling snack.

Beans

Beans are a great source of what is called a resistant starch. Most starches, like sugar, breads, and fruit juices, are digested and absorbed in the small intestine very quickly. Resistant starches, however, resist digestion and pass through to the large intestine, where they behave like dietary fibers. This keeps you feeling full longer. They are high in protein and fiber and low in carbohydrates. Eating beans will give you energy. They are an excellent health food. Below are my favorite beans.

Black Beans

Black beans are an excellent source of fiber and protein. Just one serving contains approximately 8 grams of fiber, 8 grams of protein, and 20 grams of carbohydrates. Compared with many other foods, they will give you an energy boost and keep you from feeling hungry. They are great in chili, salads, salsas, and even for breakfast.

Lentils

Lentils are also nutritional powerhouses. A serving contains 8 grams of fiber, 9 grams of protein, and 21 grams of carbohydrates, but contains virtually no fat. They will fill you up, not out. Lentils also cook quickly. Use them in soups, salads, or on their own for a delicious meal.

Dark Leafy Greens

Dark leafy greens like arugula, kale, Swiss chard, and spinach are filled with vitamins A and C, calcium, and iron. They are high in fiber and low in calories, making them great for weight loss. Make sure you buy organic greens, as they made the dirty dozen list (pg 40). You will find many delicious recipes for greens later in this book, like shakes, sautéed greens, soups, and stir fries. Give them a try. You can also eat as much as you want and not worry about gaining weight.

Blueberries

Blueberries are super high in powerful antioxidants, including vitamin C and manganese. Manganese plays an important role in converting proteins, carbohydrates, and fats into energy. Buy fresh or frozen, organic or wild.

Sweet Potatoes

Substitute sweet potatoes for white potatoes. Sweet potatoes offer many more antioxidants and nutrients per serving compared to white ones. They are also a strong anti-inflammatory, high in vitamin A, and are a low glycemic food, which helps control blood sugar.

Wild Alaskan Salmon

Wild Alaskan salmon is very high in omega-3 fatty acids and monounsaturated fats. This salmon is a lean protein that will help you lose weight. Wild Alaskan salmon can be purchased fresh in season or frozen out of season. Look for the King, Sockeye, and Coho varieties.

Green Tea

From improving brain and heart health to stress relief, green tea should become your new beverage of choice. In the past 20 years, thousands of studies [8] have shown green tea's benefits. It's excellent for weight loss since it can help increase your metabolism so you burn more calories. Studies show that green tea can also help you keep the weight off once you've lost it. What's not to love?

Physical # 2

12 months after starting the *Rehealth Yourself* plan:

I was excited and yet a little scared to be going back to the doctor's office for my annual physical and cholesterol test. I knew I had been eating healthy and exercising, but I kept wondering whether my results would be better than my last physical and cholesterol tests. Maybe my last test results were just a fluke. Maybe there was a mistake. I knew my weight had leveled out at 156. The nurse called me into the office and checked my weight and my blood pressure, which were both excellent.

I met with my doctor and discussed how I had been feeling, what I had been eating, and how I had been exercising. The doctor told me everything looked great, and he needed to check my cholesterol tests. I went to the lab and I had my blood drawn. The next day I received an email from my doctor.

To my surprise, he said, "John, your cholesterol numbers are in the acceptable range, in fact they are great! Your HDL has improved, your LDL, VDL and triglycerides have all continued to decrease from your last lipid profile. Keep up the good work." I looked at my results: My total cholesterol was down 20%, HDL up 15%, LDL down 30%, VDL down 36%, and triglycerides down an outstanding 40%.

I thought back over the last year. I knew the only changes I had made were eating healthy and exercising. I thought about some of the food I had stopped eating, and the junior cheeseburgers came to mind. I would have consumed over 250 of them over the last year if I had continued! I'm sure that had something to do with my improved health.

Chapter 5

The Grocery Store:
How to Shop for Healthy Food

"Life itself is the proper binge."

Julia Child

I enjoy grocery shopping. That's the chef in me. I'm always looking for the best healthy natural ingredients that I can find, and I do that by reading labels thoroughly.

Reading Labels

On a label [9], ingredients are listed in order of the greatest amount to the least. When I read a label, I'm looking for a few things to decide if I want to purchase the product. First, I want to see very few ingredients, preferably only 2 or 3 at most. For example, the ingredients in organic black beans should be black beans and maybe a little bit of salt. I will not buy food products if they have any preservatives, nitrates, sulfites, BHA, BHT, sodium benzoate, or any other unnatural product listed as an ingredient. If you don't know what an ingredient is or can't pronounce it, research the ingredient and find out what it is. Food companies have gotten pretty good at disguising these ingredients, so don't believe everything you read on the front of the package. CSPI (Center for Science in the Public Interest) [10] has some great information on food additives. Learn about "Chemical Cuisine" on their website. Just remember it is better to look for fewer ingredients with nothing artificial when purchasing your food products. Ideally, you will want to replace any food that is questionable with fresh, natural whole foods without labels. Fresh green beans or vine ripened tomatoes do not come with a nutrition label or a list of ingredients. If you decide to buy foods with labels, make sure you read them thoroughly.

When you are at the grocery store, look at what other people are buying. When you really stop and look, you will be amazed at what you see. I sometimes look at the ratio of "bad" food to "healthy" food in other people's carts while in the checkout aisle. Many of these consumers are overweight. This will be a great source of motivation for you. You will know the right foods to buy that will help you get healthy and lose weight naturally. It is easy to fall into this unhealthy trap and buy heavily processed, prepared foods. We are all busy, but we must take the time to fuel our bodies correctly, and simple recipes can be prepared in no time. Stick with the ingredients below and you will "rehealth yourself" quickly and naturally.

Proteins

When purchasing proteins, stick with items such as grass-fed beef and pork, organic or free-range chicken [11], and wild or organic seafood. These products should be minimally processed and 100% all natural and/or organic. Don't buy proteins with additives like nitrates, BHA, BHT, sulfites, MSG, hydrolyzed protein, or natural flavorings. This is extremely important, because some of these additives have been shown to cause problems like high blood pressure and an increased risk of cancer.

Products that usually have these additives are lunch/deli meats, hot dogs, sausages, marinated or injected products with some kind of enhancing solution, and pre-cooked meats or entrees. Do not buy anything sold as juicy, tender, extra moist, etc. Most of these products have been injected with a sodium solution that stays in the meat after cooking. First, you are paying for salt water and chemicals, and second, the food you are eating is now processed and the meat has a much higher sodium content. You must read every label on the package of meat that you pick up.

Fish and Seafood

Consuming fish and seafood is one of the very best things to do for your health. There are many types of fish and seafood, and I recommend eating a wide variety. When buying fish and seafood, look for wild, organic, or 100% all-natural fresh or frozen products. It is very important to read labels when buying fish and seafood. At the fish counter, ask the origin of the fresh fish or seafood. Ask if it is 100% natural. Many fish and seafood items will be marked "previously frozen," so ask questions.

Did you know that wild Alaskan cod can be produced in China? Cod is caught in Alaska, frozen at sea, and sent to China. The fish is then thawed, soaked or treated with sodium tripolyphosphate (STPP), cut into portions or filets, and then sent back to the USA. The box will be marked "Wild Alaskan Cod" and on a small corner of the box it will say "Produced in China." The cod now has an ingredients list, and it is not the only fish this is being done to. I have seen this with halibut, haddock, pollock, salmon, shrimp, and many other fish and seafood items. Avoid fish or seafood products from China or any other country that contain STPP as an ingredient.

Products soaked or enhanced with STPP will make the product maintain moisture or hold water, can have a preserving effect, and has a high sodium content. Check for seafood products labeled "dry," which means they have not been contaminated with STPP. Food products labeled "wet" have usually been treated with STPP. Sodium tripolyphosphate is also used in household cleaners and detergents, so it is not something I want to be consuming.

Fruits & Vegetables

Vegetables are a very important part of rehealthing yourself and losing weight, and thankfully there is a huge variety to choose from. Don't be afraid to try new vegetables or give a second chance to a vegetable you didn't like as a kid. Eating a full rainbow spectrum of colors is important, keeping in mind the darker the vegetable, the more nutrients are present.

Whenever possible, always prepare and cut whole, fresh vegetables. This really does not take more than a minute or two, but if time is a major factor and you can't cut fresh vegetables each night, then I recommend buying precut fresh vegetables. Most grocery stores now sell fresh-cut vegetables in many varieties, from diced celery, onions, and sweet peppers to combinations of asparagus and mushrooms. If you can't find pre-cut organic vegetables [12], at least make sure there are no additives, seasonings, salt, or marinades added to the vegetables.

Grocery stores are doing a better job of providing fresh, natural foods, so don't be afraid to ask for something special. You probably won't be the only one looking for these products, and stores are more likely to stock items that consumers request. As I mentioned in Chapter 3, try to buy local or organic products whenever possible. These products will be fresher and handled less. Support your local farmer! If you live near a farmer's market, buying produce from there is a great way to make connections with farmers in your area.

Below is a list of fruits and vegetables with the highest and lowest potential amounts of pesticides. For additional information, visit the Environmental Working Group website at www.ewg.org [13]. The Environmental Working Group is a non-profit American environmental organization that specializes in research and advocacy. The fruits and vegetables listed in the highest category, also known as the "dirty dozen," should be avoided as much as possible unless they have been organically grown.

Pesticide Levels of Fruit:

Highest levels of pesticides	*Lowest levels of pesticides*
Apples	Cantaloupes
Grapes	Grapefruit
Nectarines	Kiwi
Peaches	Mangoes
Strawberries	Pineapple
Cherries	

Pesticide Levels of Vegetables:

Highest levels of pesticides	*Lowest levels of pesticides*
Celery	Asparagus
Spinach	Avocados
Tomatoes	Cabbage
Cucumbers	Corn
Peppers	Eggplant
Potatoes	Mushrooms
Greens (arugula, chards, kale, etc.)	Onions
Squash (summer, yellow, and zucchini)	Sweet Peas
	Sweet Potatoes

Migraines and Preservatives

When my daughter Nicole was 16 years old, she began getting headaches quite frequently. She would notice changes to her vision, and then 15 minutes later, an intense, very painful headache would start. These headaches made it very difficult to focus at school. She tried taking ibuprofen and Tylenol but said they did almost nothing to help the pain.

We decided to go see a doctor. After several pokes, pricks, and tests, the doctor explained that Nicole was probably experiencing migraine headaches. The doctor wanted her to start taking medicine on a daily basis as a preventative therapy to help with these headaches. The doctor also prescribed a very powerful form of ibuprofen to take when she would get these headaches. When we picked up the prescriptions, we started to read the common side effects: vision problems, uncontrolled rolling of the eyes, memory problems, dizziness, confusion, burning, tingling, unusual tiredness, weakness, and many more. This medicine was only meant to treat the migraines, not cure them.

After a brief discussion, we decided that maybe a more natural approach would be a better option. We started to research migraine headaches and triggers. Preservatives and additives in food kept appearing. We started to look at Nicole's diet and eliminated all preservatives and additives like BHT, nitrites, nitrates, natural flavor, caramel color, MSG, sulfites, disodium guanylate, disodium inosinate, and yeast extract—basically any ingredient that we could not pronounce or did not know. Many of these ingredients are found in hot dogs, lunch meats, canned soups, and frozen entrees.

Nicole started to eat more healthy, natural foods, and amazingly, the migraines went away. She only gets a migraine now when she doesn't watch what she eats.

Is it really that simple to "rehealth yourself"? I believe so.

Chapter 6

The Food Plan

"The food you eat in private shows up in public."

Anonymous

Now that you have eliminated unhealthy foods and weight retention products from your daily life, you will learn how to use my system to naturally improve your health and lose weight. To make things easy, I have created a sample menu for the first week. To start, you will follow my simple 7-day meal plan. At the end of the initial 7-day plan, you can begin to swap foods from the recipes listed in the cookbook in Chapter 7 in the following week.

This process will help you form a habit of eating healthy foods. A new lifestyle of eating will be developed gradually. You will no longer crave the white processed foods that are unhealthy for you.

As you begin the meal plan, follow your menus very carefully and try not to eat anything additional. Be especially careful not to grab a bite of a cookie or a few chips. Do not allow yourself to say "It's just a couple bites of cake" or "It's just a little donut." By following this simple plan, you will get healthy and lose weight. It will be fun and very rewarding to step on the scale and watch your excess weight disappear. Once you begin to see results, you will want to continue. You'll love when your clothes become baggy, and I highly recommend donating any clothes that don't fit you any longer.

Time to Eat

Today's lifestyle has created quite a lot of stress. We work all day, fight traffic to get home, and then need to make dinner. It is very easy to just give up and go buy some fast food at the drive-through. If you find that you do not have time to make the following recipes for dinner, try some of these methods to help you create healthy meals on those stressful days. You can make delicious, healthy meals in less than 30 minutes. Here are some tips:

Plan your meals ahead of time. Once your kitchen is organized, plan your meals each week. Go to the grocery and buy everything you will need for a week. It is much less stressful knowing what you are having for dinner each night instead of waiting until the last minute.

Cook in advance. When you cook, make extra food and stock your freezer full so that you can thaw, heat, and serve when needed. Grill extra chicken breast, make a large pot of soup, roast a larger piece of meat. Any of these items can be quickly thawed and served with some fresh or frozen vegetables for a quick dinner.

Make cooking a family affair. Getting your family involved in preparing dinner also teaches them about healthy eating. Instead of everyone coming home from school or work and watching TV or playing games on the tablet, ask them to help out. Depending on the age of your kids, start with simple tasks like setting the table and filling glasses of water. Soon they'll want to do more, from cutting vegetables to making the salad to learning about the seasonings for the roasted turkey breast. You will be amazed at the amount of self-esteem helping cook the family meal can provide. Do not make cooking in the kitchen or cleaning up afterwards a chore. Instead, make it part of their daily life and they will learn how to eat healthy and make good choices.

The Meal Plan
Recipes for foods contained in the plan are in Chapter 7

Special note:

When you are scheduled to eat eggs for breakfast, use the recipes that are listed or add some of your own favorite vegetables. When a salad is scheduled, top with the ingredients listed or add your own favorite vegetables. For the beverages, try to drink green tea every day. The amount of water listed in the sample plan is the minimum you should be drinking. You can also add seltzer water or coconut water, but remember, no added sugar.

About the food, if you are not sure whether to buy organic or traditional food, refer back to chapter 5 The Grocery Store, How to Shop for Healthy Food page 36.

Measurements and Abbreviations:

oz = ounce
lb = pound
tsp = teaspoon
tbsp = tablespoon
EVOO= Extra-virgin olive oil

Day 1

Breakfast
Chocolate Mocha Protein Shake, pg 59
1 cup 50/50 coffee or green tea
12 oz filtered ice water

Morning Snack
¼ cup walnuts
1 apple
12 oz filtered ice water

Lunch
Turkey, Avocado, and Roasted Red Pepper Salad, pg 81
12 oz filtered ice water

Afternoon Snack
1 tbsp *All Natural Hummus, pg 94*
6 each carrot and celery sticks
12 oz filtered ice water

Dinner
Almond-Crusted Chicken Breast, pg 141
½ cup smashed yams, pg 123
1 cup sautéed asparagus and mushrooms, pg 120
1 cup decaf green tea
12 oz filtered ice water

Day 2

Breakfast
Very Berry Protein Shake, pg 58
1 cup 50/50 coffee or green tea
12 oz filtered ice water

Morning Snack
1 hard-boiled egg, pg 62
12 oz filtered ice water

Lunch
Grilled Chicken Salad 1, pg 70
12 oz filtered ice water

Afternoon Snack
¼ cup almonds, pumpkin seeds, and peanuts
12 oz filtered ice water

Dinner
Wild Salmon with Sautéed Veggies, pg 126
2 cups mixed green salad, pg 68
1 tbsp oriental dressing, pg 89
1 cup decaf green tea
12 oz filtered ice water

Day 3

Breakfast
Soft Scrambled Eggs with Vegetable Blast, pg 66
1 cup 50/50 coffee or green tea
12 oz filtered ice water

Morning Snack
1 tbsp *Roasted Red Pepper Hummus, pg 97*
½ cup broccoli florets
12 oz filtered ice water

Lunch
Quinoa Tabouleh with Grilled Chicken, pg 69
12 oz filtered ice water

Afternoon Snack
6 each carrots and celery sticks
12 oz filtered ice water

Dinner
Herb and Pecan Crusted Pork Tenderloin, pg 153
½ cup roasted cauliflower, pg 113
2 cups mixed green salad, pg 68, with ¼ cup raw rainbow vegetables
pg 110
1 tbsp creamy Italian dressing, pg 88
1 cup decaf green tea
12 oz filtered ice water

Day 4

Breakfast
Energize Me Shake, pg 55
1 cup 50/50 coffee or green tea
12 oz filtered ice water

Morning Snack
1 apple
12 oz filtered ice water

Lunch
1 ½ cups *12-Way Roasted Vegetable Soup, pg 104*
12 oz filtered water

Afternoon Snack
¼ cup mixed nuts, almonds, cashews, and walnuts
12 oz filtered ice water

Dinner
Grilled Balsamic Grass-Fed Sirloin Steak, pg 148
½ cup sweet potato home fries, pg 124
1 cup fresh asparagus, steamed
½ cup chef fruit salad, pg 77
1 cup decaf green tea
12 oz filtered ice water

Day 5

Breakfast
Chocolate Banana Protein Shake, pg 53
1 cup 50/50 coffee or green tea
12 oz filtered ice water

Morning Snack
1 tbsp all natural peanut butter
6 each carrot and celery sticks
12 oz filtered ice water

Lunch
White Chicken Chili, pg 107
12 oz filtered ice water

Afternoon Snack
1 tbsp *Avocado Chili Pepper Hummus, pg 95*
½ cup broccoli
12 oz filtered ice water

Dinner
Shrimp Scampi, pg 128
½ cup wild mushroom quinoa, pg 122
1 cup roasted vegetables, pg 110
2 cups mixed green salad, pg 68, topped with 3-4 grape tomatoes and
¼ cup cucumbers, diced
1 tbsp creamy Italian dressing, pg 88
1 cup decaf green tea
12 oz filtered water

Day 6

Breakfast
Asparagus, Basil, and Tomato Omelet, pg 63
1 cup 50/50 coffee or green tea
12 oz filtered ice water

Morning Snack
1 apple
12 oz filtered ice water

Lunch
Chef's Deli Salad, pg 80
12 oz filtered ice water

Afternoon Snack
¼ cup pumpkin seeds, pg 102
12 oz filtered ice water

Dinner
Chicken Breast Marsala, pg 138
2/3 cup cauliflower mash, pg 114
1 cup sautéed rainbow vegetables, pg 110
2 cups mixed green salad, pg 68
1 tbsp Italian dressing, pg 85
½ cup fresh blueberries and strawberries
1 cup decaf green tea
12 oz filtered ice water

Day 7

Breakfast
Strawberry Banana Protein Shake, pg 57
1 cup 50/50 coffee or green tea
12 oz filtered ice water

Morning Snack
1 hard-boiled egg, pg 62
12 oz filtered ice water

Lunch
Albacore Tuna Salad, pg 78
12 oz filtered ice water

Afternoon Snack
8 each carrots and celery sticks
1 tbsp almond butter
12 oz filtered ice water

Dinner
BBQ Beef Brisket, pg 149
1 cup flash fried green beans, pg 119
½ cup sweet potato fries, pg 125
2 cups mixed green salad, pg 68, topped with 4-5 cherry tomatoes
and ¼ cup sliced cucumbers
1 tbsp balsamic dressing, pg 84
1 cup decaf green tea
12 oz filtered ice water

Chapter 7

The Recipes

**"The most difficult thing is the decision to act,
the rest is merely tenacity."**

Amelia Earhart

About the food; if you are not sure whether to buy organic or traditional food, refer back to chapter 5 The Grocery Store, How to Shop for Healthy Food page 36.

Measurements and Abbreviations

oz = ounce
lb = pound
tsp = teaspoon
tbsp = tablespoon
EVOO= Extra-virgin olive oil

Breakfast

Protein Shakes

For the protein powder, I like plain or vanilla "NutriBiotic Organic Rice Protein Powder." It has a low sugar content (less than 2 grams) and low carbohydrates (less than 2 grams). There are many other protein powders available as well. Look for organic, low sugar, and low carbohydrates.

Chocolate Banana Protein Shake

Step 1:
¾ cup almond milk or coconut milk, unsweetened
¼ cup Greek yogurt, plain
½ small banana, more green than yellow
4 baby carrots
2 tsp chia seeds
1 tbsp raw cocoa, unsweetened
½ cup mixed greens (kale, Swiss chard, spinach)

Add all ingredients to blender and blend until very smooth.

Step 2:
½ cup ice
1 tbsp brown rice protein powder

Add protein powder and ice and blend until smooth. You can add more ice or almond milk depending on your desired consistency. Makes 1 serving.

Super Green Protein Shake

Step 1:
¾ cup almond milk or coconut milk, unsweetened
¼ cup Greek yogurt, plain
¼ ripe avocado, peeled, pitted, and cut into ½ inch chunks
2 tsp chia seeds
½ cup baby kale
2 dates

Add all ingredients to blender and blend until very smooth.

Step 2:
½ cup ice
1 tbsp brown rice protein powder

Add protein powder and ice and blend until smooth. You can add more ice or almond milk depending on your desired consistency. Makes 1 serving.

Energize Me Protein Shake

Step 1:
¾ cup almond milk, unsweetened
½ banana more green than yellow
¼ cup blueberries
½ cup mixed greens (kale, Swiss chard, spinach)
1 tbsp chia seeds
⅛ cup walnuts
4 baby carrots
¼ cup Greek yogurt, plain

Add all ingredients to blender and blend until very smooth.

Step 2:
½ cup ice
1 tbsp flax seed, ground
1 tbsp brown rice protein powder

Add protein powder, flax, and ice and blend until smooth. You can add more ice or almond milk depending on your desired consistency. Makes 1 serving.

Power Protein Shake

Step 1:
¾ cup almond milk or coconut milk, unsweetened
¼ cup Greek yogurt, plain
¼ ripe avocado, peeled, pitted and cut into ½ inch chunks
2 tsp chia seeds
2 tsp hemp seeds, ground
1 tbsp almond butter
2 dates
1 tbsp lentils, cooked
1 tsp cinnamon

Add all ingredients to blender and blend until very smooth.

Step 2:
½ cup ice
1 tbsp flax seed, ground
1 tbsp brown rice protein powder

Add protein powder, flax, and ice and blend until smooth. You can add more ice or almond milk depending on your desired consistency. Makes 1 serving.

Strawberry Banana Protein Shake

Step 1:
¾ cup almond milk or coconut milk, unsweetened
¼ cup Greek yogurt, plain
½ banana, more green than yellow
¼ cup organic strawberries, sliced
2 tsp chia seeds
½ cup mixed greens (kale, Swiss chard, spinach)

Add all ingredients to blender and blend until very smooth.

Step 2:
½ cup ice
1 tbsp brown rice protein powder

Add protein powder and ice and blend until smooth. You can add more ice or almond milk depending on your desired consistency. Makes 1 serving.

Very Berry Protein Shake

Step 1:
¾ cup almond milk, unsweetened
¼ cup Greek yogurt, plain
¼ cup blueberries
¼ cup strawberries (you can also use blackberries or raspberries)
2 tsp chia seeds
½ cup mixed greens (kale, Swiss chard, spinach)

Add all ingredients to blender and blend until very smooth.

Step 2:
½ cup ice
1 tbsp brown rice protein powder

Add protein powder and ice and blend until smooth. You can add more ice or almond milk depending on your desired consistency. Makes 1 serving.

Chocolate Mocha Protein Shake

Step 1:
¾ cup almond milk, unsweetened
¼ cup Greek yogurt, plain
½ banana, more green than yellow
2 tsp chia seeds
1 date
1 tbsp raw cocoa, unsweetened
2 tsp instant coffee, decaf
½ cup mixed greens (kale, Swiss chard, spinach)

Add all ingredients to blender and blend until very smooth.

Step 2:
½ cup ice
1 tbsp brown rice protein powder

Add protein powder and ice and blend until smooth. You can add more ice or almond milk depending on your desired consistency. Makes 1 serving.

Vanilla Blueberry Protein Shake

Step 1:
¾ cup almond milk, unsweetened
¼ cup Greek yogurt, plain
½ cup blueberries
2 tsp chia seeds
½ tsp vanilla extract
½ cup mixed greens (kale, Swiss chard, spinach)

Add all ingredients to blender and blend until very smooth.

Step 2:
½ cup ice
1 tbsp brown rice protein powder

Add protein powder and ice and blend until smooth. You can add more ice or almond milk depending on your desired consistency. Makes 1 serving.

Hawaiian Slim Protein Shake

Step 1:
¾ cup coconut milk, unsweetened
¼ cup pineapple, fresh or frozen, golden
½ banana, more green than yellow
2 tsp chia seeds
½ cup mixed fresh kale

Add all ingredients to blender and blend until very smooth.

Step 2:
½ cup ice
1 tbsp brown rice protein powder

Add protein powder and ice and blend until smooth. You can add more ice or almond milk depending on your desired consistency. Makes 1 serving.

Eggs

Hard-Boiled Eggs

In medium sauce pot, gently place eggs and cover with cold water. Bring water to a low simmer and cook for 12-14 minutes. Chill eggs in cool water before refrigerating.

Egg Soufflé in a Minute

1 coffee cup, microwave safe
1 egg, all natural or organic
1 tbsp uncured bacon, ham, or sausage, cooked and chopped
1 tsp onion, minced
1 tsp sweet peppers, minced
1 tbsp organic spinach, chopped

Place egg in coffee cup and mix well with a fork. Add remaining ingredients and mix. Place in microwave and cook on high for 30 seconds. Remove from microwave and mix well. Place back in microwave and cook an additional 30 seconds. If eggs are still a little runny, microwave for 10 more seconds. Be careful not to overcook the eggs or they will be tough and chewy. Season with a pinch of sea salt and fresh cracked pepper and serve.

Asparagus, Basil, and Tomato Omelet

2 eggs, all-natural or organic
1 tbsp EVOO
¼ cup asparagus, cut into ½ inch pieces, steamed for 1 minute
1 tbsp basil, minced
3 slices roma tomato
Sea salt and fresh cracked pepper to taste

It is easier to make an omelet in a non-stick pan. Use a heat-resistant rubber spatula so it doesn't melt.

Crack the eggs into a mixing bowl and mix well. Heat a non-stick sauté pan over medium-low heat. Add the EVOO. Add the eggs to the pan. Let the eggs cook for up to a minute or until the bottom starts to set. With the spatula, gently push one edge of the egg into the center of the pan, while tilting the pan to allow the still liquid egg to flow in underneath. Repeat with the other edges, until there's no liquid left. Your eggs should now resemble a pancake, which should easily slide around on the non-stick surface. If it sticks at all, loosen it with your spatula. Gently flip the omelet over, using your spatula if necessary. Cook for another few seconds, or until there is no uncooked egg left. Add the asparagus, basil and tomato on top of omelet, off to one side. Season with the sea salt and black pepper. With your spatula, lift one edge of the egg and fold it across, so that the edges line up. Cook for another minute. Gently transfer the omelet to a warm plate. Serves 1.

Texas Omelet

2 eggs, all-natural or organic
1 tbsp EVOO
2 chef sausage patties, diced
1 tbsp onions, diced
1 tbsp peppers, diced
1 tbsp mushrooms, diced
1 tsp hot sauce (optional)
Sea salt and fresh cracked pepper to taste

It is easier to make an omelet in a non-stick pan. Use a heat-resistant rubber spatula so it doesn't melt.

Crack the eggs into a mixing bowl and mix well. Heat a non-stick sauté pan over medium-low heat. Add the EVOO. Add the sausage, onions and peppers and cook for 2 minutes. Remove from pan. Add the eggs to the pan. Let the eggs cook for up to a minute or until the bottom starts to set. With the spatula, gently push one edge of the egg into the center of the pan, while tilting the pan to allow the still liquid egg to flow in underneath. Repeat with the other edges, until there's no liquid left. Your eggs should now resemble a pancake, which should easily slide around on the non-stick surface. If it sticks at all, loosen it with your spatula. Gently flip the omelet over, using your spatula to ease it over if necessary. Cook for another few seconds, or until there is no uncooked egg left. Add the sausage, onions, peppers, and mushrooms on top of omelet off to one side. Season with the sea salt and black pepper. With your spatula, lift one edge of the egg and fold it across, so that the edges line up. Cook for another minute. Gently transfer the omelet to a warm plate. Top with hot sauce and serve. Serves 1.

Soft Scrambled Eggs with Vegetable blast

2 eggs, all-natural or organic
1 tbsp EVOO
1 tbsp onion, diced
1 tbsp peppers, diced
¼ cup broccoli, cut into small florets
1 tbsp sun dried tomatoes, diced
½ cup spinach
Sea salt and fresh cracked pepper to taste

It is easier to make scrambled eggs in a non-stick pan. Use a heat-resistant rubber spatula so it doesn't melt.

Crack the eggs into a mixing bowl and mix well. Heat a non-stick sauté pan over medium-low heat. Add the EVOO. Add all vegetables except spinach and cook for 1-2 minutes. Add the eggs to the pan. As the eggs begin to cook, gently pull eggs across pan with the spatula. Continue cooking, lifting and folding eggs until no visible liquid remains. Add spinach and cook for 1 minute. Season the eggs with sea salt and black pepper. Serves 1.

Soft Scrambled Eggs with Artichokes, Smoked Salmon, and Chives

2 eggs, all-natural or organic
1 tbsp EVOO
¼ cup artichokes, diced
¼ cup smoked wild salmon, diced
2 tsp fresh chives, minced
Sea salt and fresh cracked pepper to taste

It is easier to make scrambled eggs in a non-stick pan. Use a heat-resistant rubber spatula so it doesn't melt.

Crack the eggs into a mixing bowl and mix well. Heat a non-stick sauté pan over medium-low heat. Add the EVOO. Add artichokes and smoked salmon and cook for 1 minute. Add the eggs to the pan. As the eggs begin to cook, gently pull eggs across pan with the spatula. Continue cooking, lifting and folding eggs until no visible liquid remains. Add chives and cook for 1 minute. Season the eggs with sea salt and black pepper. Serves 1.

Chef's Breakfast Sausage Patties

½ lb ground turkey
½ lb ground pork
1 tbsp fresh lemon juice
2 tsp lemon zest
¼ cup almond meal
¾ tsp sage
½ tsp ginger
1 tsp sea salt
1 tsp freshly cracked pepper
½ cup filtered water
1 tbsp EVOO

In a bowl, combine all ingredients except EVOO and mix well. Cover and refrigerate for 1 hour. Heat sauté pan to medium with EVOO. With a 1 oz scooper, portion sausage and place in sauté pan. With a spatula, press down on sausage to about ½ inch thick. Cook for 7-8 minutes, browning on both sides. Serve hot. Refrigerate or freeze remaining sausage patties.

Salads

Mixed Green Salad

Wash and gently toss equal parts of organic arugula, romaine lettuce, and spring mix. Top with your favorite raw vegetables. Use only 1 tablespoon of dressing.

Southwest Style Shrimp and Black Bean Salad

½ can black beans
½ cup sweet corn, fresh or frozen
1 avocado, ripe, peeled, pitted and cut into ½ inch chunks
½ cup tomato, diced
¼ cup green onion, diced
2 tbsp salsa, no sugar added
2 tbsp balsamic vinegar
3 tbsp EVOO
1 tsp garlic powder
Sea salt and freshly cracked pepper to taste
3 oz steamed shrimp, wild, all-natural, chilled (grilled chicken, steak, or turkey can also be substituted for the shrimp)
4 cups mixed green salad

Drain beans and rinse well with water. In a large bowl, combine all vegetables. Mix well. Add salsa, balsamic vinegar, and EVOO. Mix well. Season with sea salt and fresh cracked pepper to taste. To serve, place ¾ cup black bean mixture on top of 2 cups of mixed green salad and top with 3 oz of steamed wild, all-natural shrimp. Serves 2.

Quinoa Tabouleh

½ cup lemon juice, freshly squeezed
¼ cup EVOO
1 tsp sea salt
½ tsp fine ground black pepper
1 cup quinoa, cooked
3 cups flat-leaf parsley, chopped fine, about 3 bunches
½ cup fresh mint leaves, finely chopped
1 pt grape tomatoes, quartered
½ cup English cucumber, diced
1 tbsp roasted red peppers, diced

In a large mixing bowl, whisk together the lemon juice, olive oil, sea salt, and pepper. Add the parsley, mint, grape tomatoes, cucumbers, roasted red peppers, and quinoa. Toss the salad gently until well mixed. Refrigerate for 1 hour before serving. You can add grilled chicken breast, steak, or even grilled fish for an excellent lunch or dinner.

Grilled Chicken Salad 1

1 lb chicken breast, boneless and skinless, grilled, chilled and diced
1 celery rib, diced
⅓ cup onion, diced
¼ cup sweet red pepper, diced
¼ cup sweet peas, fresh or frozen
1 tbsp Madeira wine or dry sherry
¼ cup Vegenaise® mayonnaise
½ fresh lemon, juiced
Sea salt and fresh cracked pepper to taste
¼ cup sliced carrots
¼ cup broccoli florets

Slice the grilled chicken breast into long thin strips, then cut crosswise into small ½ inch pieces and place in a medium bowl. To the bowl, add vegetables, Vegenaise® or vegetarian mayonnaise, wine, lemon juice, salt, and pepper. Mix gently. Refrigerate. To serve, place 4-5 oz grilled chicken salad on 2 cups mixed green salad and top with sliced carrots and broccoli florets. Serves 4.

Grilled Chicken Salad 2

1 chicken breast, boneless and skinless, grilled, chilled and diced
¼ cup artichoke hearts, quartered
¼ cup olives, sliced
¼ cup roasted red peppers, sliced
1 tbsp sliced almonds
2 cups mixed greens
1 tbsp Italian dressing, pg 85

To serve, place greens on plate and top with artichokes, olives, roasted red peppers, almonds, and grilled chicken. Drizzle with Italian dressing. Serves 1.

Tex Mex Salad with Grilled Chicken

1 chicken breast, boneless and skinless, grilled, chilled and diced
¼ cup tomatoes, diced
¼ avocado, diced
2 tbsp sweet corn, fresh or frozen
¼ cup black beans
1 tbsp scallions, chopped
2 cups mixed greens
1 tbsp lime juice
2 tbsp EVOO
½ tsp chili powder
Sea salt and fresh cracked pepper to taste

To serve, in a small bowl mix lime juice, EVOO, chili powder, salt and pepper. Place greens on plate and top with remaining ingredients. Drizzle with dressing and serve. Serves 1.

Tomato Lentil Salad

1 large tomato, cut into ½ inch chunks
1 English cucumber, cut into ½ inch chunks
½ cup scallions, chopped fine
2 cups red lentils, cooked
2 cups green lentils, cooked
2 garlic cloves, minced
1 tbsp fresh cilantro, chopped
1 tbsp fresh basil, chopped
Juice from 2 lemons
1 tbsp balsamic vinegar, pg 84
½ cup EVOO
Sea salt and freshly cracked pepper to taste

Combine all vegetables and beans into a large mixing bowl. Mix balsamic vinegar, lemon juice, and EVOO together and add to vegetables. Toss gently and season with sea salt and freshly cracked pepper. Serve chilled. To serve, place ½ cup tomato lentil salad on top of 2 cups mixed green salad. Serves 4.

Greek Chicken Salad

1 chicken breast, boneless and skinless, grilled, chilled and diced
1 large tomato, cut into ½ inch chunks
½ cup red onion, sliced thin
¼ cup kalamata olives
1 tbsp feta cheese
1 tbsp balsamic dressing, pg 84
 Sea salt and freshly cracked pepper to taste

To serve, place ingredients on top of 2 cups mixed green salad.
Drizzle with balsamic dressing. Serves 1.

Cajun Cobb Salad

1 chicken breast, boneless and skinless
1 tsp cajun seasoning
1 large tomato, cut into ½ inch chunks
½ cup green beans, blanched (placed in boiling water for 10 seconds then chilled)
1 hard boiled egg, peeled, cut in ½
1 tbsp creamy Italian dressing, pg 88
 Sea salt and freshly cracked pepper to taste

Season chicken breast with the Cajun seasoning. Grill or bake chicken then chill and cut into ½ inch cubes. To serve, place ingredients on top of 2 cups mixed green salad. Drizzle with creamy Italian dressing. Serves 1.

Asian Chicken Salad

1 chicken breast, boneless and skinless, grilled, chilled and diced
¼ cup carrots, shredded
¼ cup snow peas, sliced thin
¼ cup edamame, cooked
¼ cup cucumbers, diced
1 tbsp cashews, crushed
1 tbsp oriental dressing, pg 89
 Sea salt and freshly cracked pepper to taste

To serve, place ingredients on top of 2 cups mixed green salad. Drizzle with oriental dressing. Serves 1.

Chef's Fruit Salad

1 fresh apple, diced
1 fresh mango, peeled and diced
½ cup fresh seedless grapes
¼ cup walnut pieces, raw
¼ cup dried cherries (all natural, no sugar added)
Juice from ½ fresh lemon

Combine all ingredients in bowl and mix well. Add lemon juice and toss gently. Serve chilled. Serves 4.

Albacore Tuna Salad

2 (5 oz) cans albacore tuna (in water)
1 celery rib, diced
2 tbsp onion, diced
2 tbsp sweet red pepper, diced
1 tbsp dill relish, all natural
3 tbsp vegetarian mayonnaise
½ fresh lemon, juiced
Sea salt and freshly cracked pepper to taste
10 fresh cherry tomatoes
½ cup sliced cucumber
4 cups mixed green salad

Drain water from tuna. Add tuna to medium sized bowl. To the bowl, add the vegetables, Vegenaise®, lemon juice, sea salt, and freshly cracked pepper. Mix gently and chill. To serve, place ¾ cup tuna salad on top of 2 cups of mixed green salad with ¼ cup sliced cucumber and 5 cherry tomatoes. Serves 2-3.

Smoked Wild Salmon Salad

8 oz hot smoked wild salmon, chopped
1 Asian pear, peeled and diced
¼ cup walnuts, toasted
8 yellow grape tomatoes
4 cups mixed green salad
2 tbsp fresh squeezed lemon juice
1 tbsp Italian parsley, chopped fine
3 tbsp EVOO
Sea salt and freshly cracked pepper to taste

In medium bowl, add lemon juice, parsley, and EVOO. Mix well. Add lettuce and toss. In a separate bowl, combine all other ingredients and gently mix. To serve, divide lettuce on two cold plates. Top with remaining ingredients. Season with sea salt and freshly cracked pepper and serve. Serves 2.

Chef's Deli Salad

2 cups mixed green salad
1 oz ham, sliced into strips
1 oz turkey, sliced into strips
1 oz salami, sliced into strips
½ cup raw rainbow vegetables
1 tbsp cucumber wasabi dressing, pg 87
Freshly cracked pepper to taste

To serve, place lettuce on plate and place deli meats on top of lettuce. Drizzle with cucumber wasabi dressing. Serves 1.

Turkey, Avocado and Roasted Red Pepper Salad

2 cups mixed green salad
3 oz roasted turkey breast, sliced
¼ avocado, peeled, pitted, and cut into ¼-inch chunks
2 tbsp roasted red peppers, diced
1 tbsp balsamic dressing, pg 84
Freshly cracked pepper to taste

To serve, place lettuce on plate and top with turkey, avocado, roasted red peppers, and onion. Drizzle with balsamic dressing. Serves 1.

Asparagus, Italian Prosciutto, and Melon Salad

6 asparagus spears, blanched (placed in boiling water for 10 seconds then chill)
4 slices Italian prosciutto
2 wedges of fresh melon, such as cantaloupe, crenshaw, or honeydew
2 cups mixed green salad
1 tbsp roasted red pepper dressing, pg 90

To serve, wrap melon with prosciutto and place on top of 2 cups of mixed green salad. Top with asparagus and drizzle with roasted red pepper dressing. Serves 1.

The "Dinner" Salad

¾ cup left over protein (chicken, pork, beef etc) from dinner, chopped
1 cup left over vegetables from dinner
1 tbsp sliced almonds, cashews, walnuts or roasted pepitas
2 cups mixed greens
1 tbsp dressing, your choice pages 84-90

To serve, place greens on plate and top with protein, vegetables and nuts. Drizzle with 1 tablespoon of your favorite dressing. Serves 1.

Dressings

Balsamic Dressing

¼ cup balsamic vinegar
¾ cup EVOO
2 cloves garlic, minced, or 1 tsp garlic powder
1 tsp sea salt
1 tsp freshly cracked pepper

Combine all ingredients in shaker. Shake well. Chill. Serving size equals 1 tablespoon. For a creamy version, blend in food processor or use hand (stick) blender.

Italian Dressing

3 tbsp freshly squeezed lemon juice
1 tbsp fresh Italian parsley, chopped fine
2 tsp Dijon mustard
1 clove garlic, minced
1 tsp oregano
½ cup EVOO
Sea salt and freshly cracked pepper to taste

Combine all ingredients in shaker. Shake well. Chill. Serving size equals 1 tablespoon.

Creamy Cucumber Dill Dressing

2 tbsp freshly squeezed lemon juice
½ cup plain Greek yogurt
¼ cup cucumbers, chopped
1 tsp fresh dill, chopped
1 clove garlic, minced
¼ cup EVOO
Sea salt and fresh cracked pepper to taste

Combine all ingredients in food processor or blender. Blend well and refrigerate. Serving size equals 1 tablespoon.

Cucumber Wasabi Dressing

2 tbsp white wine vinegar
1 tsp fresh Italian parsley, chopped fine
½ cup plain Greek yogurt
¼ cup cucumbers, chopped
2 tsp wasabi paste
¼ cup EVOO
Sea salt and freshly cracked pepper to taste

Combine all ingredients in food processor or blender. Blend well and refrigerate. Serving size equals 1 tablespoon.

Creamy Italian Dressing

2 tbsp freshly squeezed lemon juice
1 tsp fresh Italian parsley, chopped fine
½ cup plain Greek yogurt
2 tsp Dijon mustard
1 clove garlic, minced
1 tsp oregano
¼ cup EVOO
Sea salt and freshly cracked pepper to taste

Combine all ingredients in shaker. Shake well. Chill. Serving size equals 1 tablespoon.

Oriental Dressing

½ cup EVOO
¼ cup rice vinegar
2 tbsp lite soy sauce
1 tsp toasted sesame oil
1 tbsp freshly squeezed orange juice
1 tbsp green onion, minced
1 tbsp almonds, toasted, ground

Combine all ingredients in shaker. Shake well. Chill. Serving size equals 1 tablespoon.

Roasted Red Pepper Dressing

3 tbsp roasted red peppers, minced
1 tsp fresh Italian parsley, chopped fine
1 clove garlic, minced
2 tbsp red wine vinegar
½ cup EVOO
Sea salt and freshly cracked pepper to taste

Combine all ingredients in food processor or blender. Blend well.
Refrigerate. Serving size equals 1 tablespoon.

Seasonings

All Purpose Seasoning

½ cup granulated garlic
1 tbsp sea salt, fine
1 tsp paprika
2 tsp dried parsley, ground

In small container add all ingredients. Place lid on container and shake well. Keep container away from heat and light for better shelf life.

Blackening or Cajun Seasoning

2 tbsp paprika
1 tbsp garlic powder
1 tbsp onion powder
2 tsp black pepper, ground
1 ½ tsp cayenne pepper
1 tsp dried oregano leaves
1 tsp dried thyme leaves
1 tsp fine sea salt

In small container add all ingredients. Place lid on container and shake well. Keep container away from heat and light for better shelf life.

Italian Seasoning

2 tbsp dried basil
2 tbsp dried oregano
2 tbsp dried rosemary, ground
1 tbsp dried marjoram
1 tbsp garlic powder
1 tbsp onion powder
1 tsp black pepper, ground
1 tsp sea salt, fine

In small container add all ingredients. Place lid on container and shake well. Keep container away from heat and light for better shelf life.

Snacks

All-Natural Hummus

1 can chick peas or garbanzo beans, drained and rinsed
1 tbsp tahini paste (optional)
Juice from 1 large fresh lemon
1 clove fresh garlic or 1 tsp of minced garlic
1 tbsp fresh parsley, chopped fine
½ cup EVOO
¼-½ cup filtered water
Sea salt and freshly cracked pepper to taste

Combine all ingredients in blender. Blend well, scraping sides until very creamy. If the hummus is too thick, add more water.

Avocado Chili Pepper Hummus

1 can chickpeas or garbanzo beans, drained and rinsed
1 tbsp tahini paste (optional)
Juice from 1 large fresh lemon
1 avocado, peeled and pitted
1 clove fresh garlic or 1 tsp of garlic powder
1 tsp fresh parsley, chopped fine
1-2 tsp red chili pepper sauce
½ cup EVOO
¼-½ cup filtered water
Sea salt and freshly cracked pepper to taste

Combine all ingredients in blender. Blend well, scraping sides until very creamy. If the hummus is too thick, add more water.

3-Bean Hummus

½ can black beans, drained and rinsed
½ can great northern beans, drained and rinsed
½ cup red lentils, cooked
1 tbsp tahini paste (optional)
Juice from 1 small fresh lemon
1 clove fresh garlic or 1 tsp of garlic powder
1 tbsp fresh parsley chopped fine
½ cup EVOO
½ cup filtered water
Sea salt and freshly cracked pepper to taste

Combine all ingredients in blender. Blend well, scraping sides until very creamy. If the hummus is too thick, add more water.

Roasted Red Pepper Hummus

1 can chickpeas or garbanzo beans, drained and rinsed
½ cup roasted red peppers
1 clove fresh garlic or 1 tsp garlic powder
¼ cup EVOO
Filtered water if needed
Sea salt and freshly cracked pepper to taste

Combine all ingredients in blender. Blend well, scraping sides until very creamy. If the hummus is too thick, add more water.

Avocado Red Pepper Deviled Eggs

6 eggs
½ avocado, peeled and pitted
1 tbsp roasted red pepper, minced fine
Juice from ½ fresh lemon
1 tbsp EVOO
1 tsp sea salt
½ tsp fresh cracked pepper
½ tsp paprika

In medium sauce pot, gently place eggs and cover with cold water. Bring water to a low simmer and cook for 12-14 minutes. Chill eggs in cool water before refrigerating.

When eggs are cool, peel and cut in half lengthwise. Gently scoop out the center yolks and place in bowl. Mash the yolks with a fork until smooth. Add the avocado, red pepper, lemon juice, EVOO, sea salt and pepper and mix well. With a tablespoon scoop the mixture and place back into the egg white halves dividing evenly. Sprinkle with paprika. Store covered in the refrigerator for up to 4 days. Enjoy as a snack or as an addition to a meal.

Jalapeno Caramelized Onion Deviled Eggs

6 eggs
1 tbsp jalapeno pepper, seeded and diced (warning, use rubber gloves during preparation)
1 tbsp caramelized onion, pg 100
Juice from ½ fresh lemon
1 tbsp EVOO
1 tsp sea salt
½ tsp fresh cracked pepper
½ tsp paprika

In medium sauce pot, gently place eggs and cover with cold water. Bring water to a low simmer and cook for 12-14 minutes. Chill eggs in cool water before refrigerating.

When eggs are cool, peel and cut in half lengthwise. Gently scoop out the center yolks and place in bowl. Mash the yolks with a fork until smooth. Add the jalapeno, caramelized onion, lemon juice, EVOO, sea salt and pepper and mix well. With a tablespoon scoop the mixture and place back into the egg white halves dividing evenly. Sprinkle with paprika. Store covered in the refrigerator for up to 4 days. Enjoy as a snack or as an addition to a meal.

Caramelized Onions

1 sweet onion, diced
1 tbsp EVOO
½ tsp sea salt

Heat a medium size pan to medium high. Add EVOO. When oil starts to shine add onions. Stir onions until well coated with oil and spread evenly over pan. Cook onions for several minutes. Do not stir onions until they are brown. Once brown stir well and repeat until onions are dark brown. Be careful not to burn the onions. Depending on your stove you may need to turn your heat to medium. Once the onions are dark brown add the sea salt and mix well. Remove from pan to cool.

Roasted nuts

To toast nuts, preheat oven to 325F. Place nuts on a baking pan and spread out evenly. Bake for about 15-20 minutes or until golden brown. Store nuts in a sealed container for freshness.

Roasted Garlic Pepitas (Pumpkin Seeds)

1 cup pepitas, raw
1 tsp coconut oil
1 tsp garlic powder
Pinch of sea salt

Place pepitas in large sauté pan. Add oil. Turn heat on medium-high. Toss and turn pepitas frequently as they start to brown and crackle. Add garlic powder and sea salt and mix well. When pepitas are browned, transfer to a cold tray to cool. Use as a snack or salad topper.

Soups

Lean and Mean Chili

2 lbs ground turkey
1 lb hot Italian turkey sausage
1 cup celery, diced
1 cup sweet onions, diced
1 can (15 oz) navy beans
1 can (15 oz) black beans
4 cloves minced garlic
2-3 tbsp EVOO
2 tbsp chili powder
1 tsp cayenne pepper
1 tsp black pepper
1 tbsp paprika
2 tsp cumin
1 tsp oregano
2 tsp garlic powder
1 tbsp sea salt
3 (16 oz) cans crushed tomatoes
1 cup dry red wine
2 quarts beef stock, low sodium

In a large stainless steel stockpot, add EVOO and meat. Cook until brown. Add garlic, onions, and celery, and cook for 3-4 minutes. Add the rest of the ingredients. Simmer for 40-50 minutes. Add more beef stock if soup is too thick. Chili can be portioned and frozen. Serves 6.

12-Way Vegetable Soup

1 cup cabbage, shredded
1 cup carrots, ½ inch diced
1 cup cauliflower, cut into 1-inch florets
1 cup celery, ½ inch diced
1 cup sweet onion, ½ inch diced
½ cup green pepper, ½ inch diced
1 cup Brussel sprouts, shredded
1 cup mushrooms, sliced
1 cup frozen sweet peas
2 large tomatoes, diced
4 cups spinach
2 cups kale, chopped
3 quarts vegetable stock, low sodium
2 tsp sea salt
2 tsp freshly cracked black pepper

In large stockpot, add 3 quarts of organic vegetable stock and all vegetables except spinach. Bring to a boil and then reduce to a simmer. Cook until vegetables are tender, about 45 minutes. Add spinach and season with sea salt and freshly cracked pepper. If the soup is too thick, add more vegetable stock. Soup can be portioned and frozen. Serves 8.

Bountiful Bean Soup

1 cup carrots, ½ inch diced
1 cup celery, ½ inch diced
1 cup sweet onion, ½ inch diced
1 can (15 oz) navy beans
1 can (15 oz) great northern beans
1 can (15 oz) light kidney beans
1 large tomato, diced
2 quarts vegetable stock, low sodium
Sea salt and freshly cracked pepper to taste

In a large stockpot, add all vegetables. Cover with 2 quarts of vegetable stock. Bring to a boil, and then reduce to a simmer. Cook until vegetables are just tender, about 30-45 minutes. Season the soup with sea salt and freshly cracked pepper. If the soup is too thick, add more vegetable stock. Soup can be portioned and frozen. Serves 6.

Black-Eyed Pea and Smoked Turkey Soup

3 cups black-eyed peas, presoaked for 24 hours in water, then
drained and rinsed
1 cup carrots, ½ inch diced
1 cup celery, ½ inch diced
1 cup sweet onion, ½ inch diced
2 cups smoked turkey breast, diced
2 cups kale, chopped
2 quarts chicken stock, low sodium
Sea salt and freshly cracked pepper to taste

In large stock pot (8 quart), add the black-eyed peas and cover with
water. Cook until tender, about 20-30 minutes. Drain water, then add
vegetables and smoked turkey. Add the chicken stock and bring to a
boil, and then reduce to a simmer. Cook until vegetables are just
tender, about 30 minutes. Add kale and cook for an additional 5
minutes or until tender. Season the soup with sea salt and freshly
cracked pepper. If the soup is too thick, add more chicken stock.
Soup can be portioned and frozen. Serves 6.

White Chicken Chili

2 cans (15 oz) great northern beans, rinsed and drained
2 cups chicken breast, boneless, skinless, diced
1 cup celery, chopped
1 cup sweet onions, chopped
4 cloves garlic, chopped
2 (4 oz) cans roasted green chilies, drained, diced
1 tbsp EVOO
1 tbsp ground cumin
2 quart chicken stock, low sodium
Sea salt and freshly cracked pepper to taste

Heat a large stock pot to medium-high. Add the EVOO, chicken, celery, onions, garlic, and chilies and cook until tender, about 5 minutes. Add remaining ingredients and simmer for 30-45 minutes, or until vegetables are tender. Carefully remove half of soup and blend in a food processor. Place pureed soup back into pot and simmer for 10 additional minutes. If the soup is too thick, add more chicken stock. Season the soup with sea salt and freshly cracked pepper. The soup can be portioned and frozen. Serves 6.

Spicy Italian Sausage and Quinoa Soup

1 lb hot Italian turkey sausage, sliced
1 cup onion, diced
1 cup celery, diced
2 cloves garlic, minced
1 tsp EVOO
2 quarts chicken stock, low sodium
1 can (15 oz) great northern beans
1 can (26 oz) tomatoes, diced
1 cup quinoa
2 cups spinach, fresh
Sea salt and freshly cracked pepper to taste

Heat a large stock pot to medium and add EVOO, sausage, onions, celery, and garlic. Cook for 10 minutes. Add broth, beans, tomatoes, and quinoa, and bring to a simmer. Cook 15-20 minutes, or until quinoa is tender. If soup is too thick, add more chicken stock. Add spinach and season with sea salt and freshly cracked pepper to taste. Soup can be portioned and frozen. Serves 6.

Beef and Lentil Soup

2 cups green or red lentils, rinsed
1 cup carrots, ½ inch diced
1 cup celery, ½ inch diced
1 cup sweet onion, ½ inch diced
2 cups beef (chuck, round, sirloin), cooked and diced
1 cup tomatoes, diced
2 quarts beef stock, low sodium
Sea salt and freshly cracked pepper to taste

In a large stockpot, add the lentils, cover with water, and cook until tender. Drain water and add vegetables. Cover with 2 quarts of beef stock. Bring to a boil and reduce to a simmer. Cook until vegetables are just tender, about 30-45 minutes. Season the soup with sea salt and fresh cracked pepper to taste. If the soup is too thick, add more beef stock. Soup can be portioned and frozen. Serves 6.

Sides / Vegetables

Rainbow Vegetables

Combine equal combinations of the following ingredients. All vegetables are diced unless noted. Vegetables can be eaten raw, pan sautéed, steamed, or oven roasted.

Broccoli (cut into small florets)
Carrots
Cauliflower (cut into small florets)
Celery
Sweet Onion
Red Pepper
Green Pepper
Mushrooms (sliced)

Beans and Greens

8 oz fresh organic greens (arugula, Swiss chard, and kale)
½ cup navy beans, cooked
½ cup black beans, cooked
¼ cup sweet onion, sliced
¼ cup sweet peppers, sliced
1 tbsp fresh garlic, minced
¼ cup vegetable stock, low sodium
1 tbsp EVOO
Salt and freshly cracked pepper to taste

Heat a large sauté pan to medium. Add EVOO, garlic, onions, and peppers. Cook for about 2-3 minutes until light brown. Add beans and cook for about 1 minute. Add greens and stock, place a lid over pan and cook for an additional 1-2 minutes. Greens should just be wilting. Season the beans and greens with sea salt and freshly cracked pepper to taste. Toss gently and serve immediately. Serves 2.

Simple Sautéed Greens

8 oz fresh organic greens (spinach, arugula, Swiss chard, kale, etc.)
1 tbsp fresh garlic, minced
1 tbsp dry white wine (optional)
1 tsp fresh lemon juice
1 tbsp EVOO
¼ cup sliced mushrooms
¼ cup diced sweet onions
Sea salt and freshly cracked pepper to taste

Heat a large sauté pan to medium. Add EVOO, garlic, mushrooms, and onions, cook for about 3 minutes until light brown. Add greens, white wine, and lemon juice. Cover with a lid and cook for 1-2 minutes. Greens should be just wilting. Season the greens with sea salt and freshly cracked pepper to taste. Serve immediately. Serves 2.

Roasted Cauliflower

2-3 cups cauliflower, washed and cut into 2-inch florets
2 tbsp coconut oil
1 tsp garlic powder
Sea salt and freshly cracked pepper

Preheat oven to 375F. Toss cauliflower with coconut oil. Season the cauliflower with garlic a pinch of sea salt, and freshly cracked pepper. Roast in oven until light brown, about 30-40 minutes. Serves 4.

Cauliflower Mash

2-3 cups cauliflower, washed and cut into 1- or 2-inch florets
1 tsp garlic powder
1 tsp chopped fresh lemon thyme
1-2 tbsp EVOO
Sea salt and freshly cracked pepper to taste

Place cauliflower in large sauce pot and cover with filtered water. Bring to a boil, and then reduce to a simmer. Cook cauliflower until tender, about 20 minutes. Drain water and place cauliflower in food processor. Add oil, garlic, and thyme. Blend until smooth. Add more EVOO if the cauliflower mash is too thick. Season the cauliflower mash with sea salt and freshly cracked pepper to taste. Serves 4.

Cauliflower "Cous Cous"

2 cups cauliflower florets
2 tbsp sweet onion, minced
1 clove garlic, minced
1 tbsp coconut oil
½ tsp sea salt
½ tsp freshly cracked black pepper

Place the cauliflower in a food processor and pulse several times until it looks like the size of peas. Heat the coconut oil in a large skillet over medium heat. Add the cauliflower, onion, and garlic and sauté, stirring frequently, until cauliflower turns light brown. Season with the sea salt and black pepper. You can also add mushrooms, broccoli (pulse with cauliflower) or diced sweet peppers. Serves 2.

Herb Zucchini Fries

2 large zucchini, cut into ¼-inch x 3-inch strips
½ cup almond meal
1 tsp garlic powder
1 tsp thyme
½ tsp rosemary
1 egg, beaten
2 tsp grape seed oil
Sea salt and freshly cracked pepper to taste

Preheat oven to 400F. Lightly grease sheet pan with grape seed oil. In a small bowl, mix all dry ingredients together. Dip zucchini into egg mixture first, then into dry ingredients and coat well. Evenly place on sheet pan. Season the zucchini with sea salt and freshly cracked pepper. Bake zucchini fries in oven about 35 minutes or until golden brown. Serves 3-4.

Balsamic Beets

2 cups red beets, cubed
1 cup balsamic vinegar
1 tsp chili pepper flakes, optional
1 tsp fresh herbs, optional

Place beets and vinegar in sauce pan. Bring to a boil and reduce heat to a simmer. Simmer beets until vinegar is reduced to about a ¼ cup. Keep refrigerated. Serve chilled on your favorite salad or as a quick snack or appetizer before your meal.

Edamame on Fire

1 cup edamame, frozen, shelled
1 tsp EVOO
1 tsp crushed hot chili peppers
½ tsp garlic powder
Sea salt and freshly cracked pepper to taste

Bring 3 cups of water to a boil, add edamame, and cook for 5 minutes. While the edamame is cooking, heat a nonstick sauté pan on low/med heat. Add the EVOO to the sauté pan. When edamame has cooked for 5 minutes, drain well and add to sauté pan. Add the chili peppers, garlic powder, and season with sea salt and freshly cracked pepper. Cook for 3 minutes, stirring frequently. Serve warm or chilled. Serves 2.

Flash-Fried French Green Beans (Haricots Verts)

1 lb French green beans (haricots verts), trimmed and washed
½ cup sweet onions, sliced thin
1 tsp fresh garlic, minced
¼ cup filtered water mixed with 1 tsp fresh lemon juice
1 tbsp grape seed oil
Salt and freshly cracked pepper to taste

Heat a sauté pan to med/high with the grape seed oil. When pan is hot, carefully add beans, onions, and garlic. Stir frequently to avoid burning. Cook vegetables until brown, about 5 minutes. Add water and lemon juice, and place lid on pan. Cook for about 2 additional minutes. Remove lid and season with salt and freshly cracked pepper to taste.
Serves 4.

Asparagus with Scallions and Woodland Mushrooms

1 lb asparagus, thin, with bottom 1 inch cut off
1 cup wild mushrooms (cremini, shiitake, oyster, etc.), sliced
1 tbsp scallions, chopped
1 tbsp EVOO
Sea salt and freshly cracked pepper to taste

Heat a medium size sauté pan over medium heat. When hot, add
EVOO and mushrooms. Cook for 2-3 minutes. Add asparagus and
scallions and cook for about 5-7 minutes, stirring occasionally.
Season with sea salt and freshly cracked pepper to taste. Serves 4.

Roasted Vegetables

1 cup broccoli, cut into 1-inch florets
1 cup cauliflower, cut into 1-inch florets
1 cup sweet onion, cut into 1-inch cubes
½ cup carrots, ½ inch diced
½ cup green pepper, cut into 1-inch cubes
½ cup squash (acorn, butternut, etc.), cut into 1-inch cubes
½ cup zucchini, cut into 1-inch cubes
½ cup mushrooms, cut into 1-inch pieces
2 tbsp EVOO
1 tsp garlic powder
Salt and freshly cracked pepper to taste

Preheat oven to 400F. In a large bowl, combine all vegetables and toss with EVOO. Place vegetables on sheet pan, spreading them out evenly. Season the vegetables with garlic powder, sea salt, and freshly cracked black pepper. Place in oven and roast until golden brown, about 30-40 minutes. Serves 4-6.

Wild Mushroom Quinoa

¼ cup sweet onion, diced
½ cup wild mushrooms, portobello, oyster or shiitake, diced
1 garlic clove, minced
1 cup quinoa
1 tbsp EVOO
2 ½ cups chicken stock, low sodium
Sea salt and freshly cracked pepper to taste

Heat a medium-sized sauce pot to medium-high. Add EVOO,
onions, and mushrooms. Cook for about 4 minutes, and then add
quinoa and chicken stock. Reduce heat, cover and bring to a simmer.
Cook quinoa until tender and stock is absorbed, about 20 minutes.
Season the quinoa with sea salt and freshly cracked pepper to taste.
Serves 4.

Smashed Yams

2 large sweet potatoes or yams, peeled and cut into ½-inch cubes
1 tbsp EVOO
Sea salt and freshly cracked pepper to taste

Place sweet potato in a stainless steel sauce pot. Cover with filtered water. Bring to a boil and reduce to a simmer. Cook until potatoes are soft and tender, about 20 minutes. Drain water. Add oil to potatoes. With hand/stick mixer, blend until smooth. If potatoes are too thick, add a little water. Season with sea salt and freshly cracked pepper to taste. Serves 4.

Sweet Potato Home Fries

2 large sweet potatoes, peeled and cut into ½-inch cubes
½ sweet onion, diced
2 tbsp coconut oil
1 tsp garlic powder
Sea salt and freshly cracked pepper to taste

Heat a non-stick sauté pan to medium-high and add coconut oil. Add onions and sweet potatoes, and place lid on pan. Reduce heat to medium. Turn onions and sweet potatoes every 4-5 minutes with spatula, being careful not to burn them. Cook until sweet potatoes are browned and just tender, about 20 minutes. Season the sweet potatoes with garlic powder, sea salt and freshly cracked pepper to taste. Serves 4.

Sweet Potato Fries

2 large sweet potatoes, peeled and cut into ¼-inch strips
1 tbsp EVOO
1 tsp garlic powder
1 tsp rosemary, minced
Sea salt and freshly cracked pepper to taste
2 tsp grape seed oil

Preheat oven to 375F. Lightly grease sheet pan with grape seed oil. In a small bowl, toss sweet potatoes in EVOO. Place sweet potatoes on sheet pan, and season with garlic powder, rosemary, sea salt, and freshly cracked pepper. Bake in oven for 35-45 minutes, turning once until crisp and golden brown. Serves 4.

Entrees

Seafood

Wild Salmon with Sautéed Veggies

4 pieces Wild King, Sockeye, Coho, or organic Atlantic salmon (6oz each)
1 cup sweet onion, diced
1 cup red sweet pepper, diced
1 cup carrots, diced
1 cup portabella mushrooms, sliced
1 cup fresh spinach
2 tbsp filtered water
Sea salt and freshly cracked pepper to taste
1 tbsp coconut oil
2 leaves fresh basil, sliced thin
2 cups brown basmati rice, cooked
4 wedges of fresh lemon

Heat oven to 350F. Season salmon with sea salt and freshly cracked pepper and place on non-stick baking sheet skin side down and place in oven. Cook until firm, about 10-15 minutes or until internal temperature reaches 145 degrees. Heat a medium size sauté pan to medium high and add the coconut oil. Add all vegetables except spinach to sauté pan and cook until tender, about 8-10 minutes. Add spinach and water. Cook until just wilted, then add basil. To serve, place ½ cup hot rice on each plate then top with vegetables. To remove skin from salmon, slide spatula in between skin and fish. Skin should come off easily. Place salmon on top of vegetables and rice. Squeeze lemon wedge over salmon. Serves 4.

Oriental Shrimp and Vegetable Stir Fry

1 lb wild shrimp, peeled and deveined with tails removed
1 cup sweet onion, sliced thin
1 cup red sweet pepper, sliced thin
1 cup carrots, sliced thin
1 cup Portobello mushrooms, sliced thin
1 cup fresh spinach
2 tbsp sesame oil
1 tbsp lite teriyaki sauce
2 tbsp filtered water
2 cups brown basmati rice, cooked

Heat a non-stick skillet to medium-high. Add sesame oil to pan. When hot, add shrimp. Cook 3 minutes, stirring frequently. Add all vegetables to sauté pan and cook until vegetables are tender, about 5 minutes. Add spinach, teriyaki sauce, and water. Cook until spinach is just wilted. To serve, place ½ cup of hot rice on each plate and top with vegetables and shrimp. Serves 4.

Shrimp Scampi

16 wild jumbo shrimp, peeled and deveined
3 cloves garlic, minced
2 tbsp coconut or grape seed oil
½ cup dry white wine
3 tbsp grass-fed butter, room temperature
Sea salt and freshly cracked pepper to taste

Preheat a large skillet to medium-high. Add coconut oil. Pat dry shrimp and add to pan. Cook shrimp about 2 minutes per side and remove from pan. Turn heat down to medium, add garlic, and cook for 1 minute. Add white wine and cook for additional 3 minutes. Add shrimp back to pan and turn heat off. Add butter and stir until mixed well. Season with sea salt and fresh cracked pepper. Serve immediately. Serve with ½ cup wild mushroom quinoa, pg 122 and roasted vegetables, pg 121. Serves 4.

Crab Cakes

1 lb crab meat
¼ cup sweet onion, diced
¼ cup red sweet pepper, diced
1 egg
1 tsp Dijon mustard
1 tbsp Vegenaise® or all-natural mayonnaise
½ cup almond meal
½ tsp sea salt
2 tsp freshly cracked pepper
2 tbsp EVOO
1 tbsp cocktail sauce, pg 163

In large bowl, combine crab and vegetables and mix well. Add egg, mustard, mayonnaise, almond meal, sea salt, and pepper and mix well. Heat a large nonstick pan to medium-high. Add EVOO. With a 2 oz scooper, form crab mixture into 2 oz balls and place in hot pan. Gently push down on crab balls to about ¾ inch thick. Cook crab cakes until just brown, about 3-5 minutes, then turn to other side and repeat. Serve with cauliflower cous cous, pg 112 and simple greens, pg 112. Serves 4.

Wild Cod Fish Fry

4 pieces wild cod loins (6 oz each)
1 egg
½ cup almond meal
½ tsp garlic powder
½ tsp celery powder
1 tsp freshly cracked pepper
1 tsp sea salt
1 tbsp grape seed oil
1 tbsp tartar sauce, pg 173

Preheat oven to 425F. In a small bowl, beat egg. In another bowl, combine all dry ingredients. Grease baking sheet with the grape seed oil. Dip cod in egg mixture and then coat heavily with dry ingredients. Place cod on baking sheet and bake in oven for 10 minutes at 425F, and then lower to 350F and bake for 10 minutes. Remove cod from oven when internal temperature reaches 155F and fork can be inserted easily. Serve with sweet potato fries, pg 125 and steamed rainbow vegetables, pg 110. Serves 4.

Coconut-Crusted Tilapia with Mango Salsa

4 pieces tilapia, (6 oz each)
½ cup shredded coconut, unsweetened
1 egg, beaten
1 tsp freshly cracked pepper
1 tsp sea salt
2 tsp coconut oil
4 tbsp mango salsa, pg 169

Preheat oven to 350F. In small bowl, combine coconut, sea salt, and pepper. Carefully dredge the tilapia in the egg mixture and then into coconut coating evenly. Use coconut oil to grease baking sheet pan. Place tilapia on baking sheet pan and place in oven. Bake until tilapia is golden brown, about 20-30 minutes or until internal temperature reaches 155F. Let rest 3-4 minutes and top with 1 tablespoon mango salsa, pg 169. Serve with ½ cup brown basmati rice and a mixed green salad, pg 68. Serves 4.

Mediterranean Roasted Halibut

4 pieces halibut, skinless and boneless (6 oz each)
2 tbsp EVOO
2 tsp shallots, minced
½ cup cherry tomatoes, cut in half
¼ cup black olives, pitted and chopped
2 tsp capers, chopped
1 tsp oregano
1 tsp fresh lemon juice
1 tsp balsamic vinegar
½ tbsp grape seed oil
1 tsp sea salt and freshly cracked pepper

Preheat oven to 450F. Rub halibut with ½ of the EVOO. Season the halibut with oregano, sea salt, and freshly cracked pepper. Grease a baking sheet with the grape seed oil. Place the halibut on baking sheet and roast in oven for about 15-20 minutes, or until internal temperature reaches 155F. While the halibut is cooking, in a sauté pan add remaining EVOO and heat to medium-high. Add shallots and cook for about 15 seconds. Add tomatoes, olives and capers, and sauté for 30 seconds. Add lemon juice and balsamic vineger and cook for an additional 2 minutes. Remove from heat and keep warm. To serve, top each piece of halibut with the Mediterranean mixture. Serve with ½ cup brown basmati rice and roasted rainbow vegetables, pg 110. Serves 4.

Ginger Soy Mahi Mahi

4 pieces mahi mahi, skinless and boneless (6 oz each)
2 tbsp light soy sauce
Juice from 1 fresh orange
1 tbsp fresh lemon juice
1 tsp sesame oil
1 cloves garlic, minced
1 tbsp ginger, peeled and minced
1 tsp red pepper flakes
2 tsp sesame seeds

Place mahi mahi in shallow glass dish. Mix all ingredients together and pour on top of mahi mahi. Let marinate for 1 hour, turning mahi mahi after 30 minutes. Preheat grill to medium-high. Cook mahi mahi on hot grill about 5-6 minutes per side or until internal temperature reaches 155F. Serve with ½ cup brown basmati rice and roasted vegetables, pg 121. Serves 4.

Blackened Sea Scallops

8 large sea scallops, chemical free (dry)
1-2 tbsp blackening seasoning
½ tbsp grape seed oil
2 lemon wedges

Lay scallops on tray and coat well with the blackening seasoning.
Heat a large sauté pan to medium high. Add the grape seed oil to
pan. Carefully add scallops to pan and cover with lid leaving slightly
ajar. Cook scallops for 3-4 minutes then using tongs carefully turn
scallops over. Cook scallops an additional 3-4 minutes. Scallops will
be done when they are white and firm. Remove scallops from pan
and serve with lemon wedge. Serve with ½ cup brown basamati rice
and steamed rainbow vegetables, pg 110. Serves 2.

Rainbow Trout Almondine

4 rainbow trout filets
1 tbsp grape seed oil
1 tsp all purpose seasoning salt
¼ cup almonds, slivered
Juice from 1 lemon
2 tbsp butter, unsalted grass fed

Lay trout on tray and season with the all purpose seasoning. Heat a large sauté pan to medium high. Add the grape seed oil to pan. Carefully add trout to pan skin side up. Cook trout 4-5 minutes. With spatula flip the trout over and cook for an additional 4-5 minutes. With a spatula remove trout from pan and keep warm. Add the almonds and lemon juice to pan and cook for about 2 minutes. Turn off heat and add butter to pan. Stir until butter is melted. With a spatula place trout skin side down on plate and top each filet with the almond mixture. Serve with ½ cup wild mushroom quinoa, pg 122 and flash fried green beans, pg 119. Serves 4.

Crab Stuffed Portobello Mushrooms

4 large portobello mushrooms 4-5 inches round, stems removed
1 tbsp EVOO
1 lb crab meat
¼ cup sweet onion, diced
¼ cup red sweet pepper, diced
1 egg
1 tsp Dijon mustard
1 tbsp Vegenaise® or all-natural mayonnaise
½ cup almond meal
1 tsp sea salt
2 tsp fresh cracked pepper
2 tbsp EVOO
1 tbsp cocktail sauce, pg 163

Heat oven to 375 degrees. Rub mushrooms with EVOO and place in baking dish. Bake mushrooms for 15 minutes. Remove from oven and cool. In large bowl, combine crab and vegetables and mix well. Add egg, mustard, mayonnaise, almond meal, sea salt, and pepper and mix well. Top the portobello mushrooms with the crab mixture dividing evenly. Place crab stuffed mushrooms in oven and bake for about 20 minutes. Serve with roasted vegetables, pg 121. Serves 4.

Poultry

Grilled Apple Cider Chicken Breast

4 pieces chicken breast, boneless and skinless
2 cloves garlic, minced
2 tbsp EVOO
1 tbsp apple cider vinegar
1 tsp freshly cracked pepper
1 tsp sea salt

Combine all ingredients in bowl and mix well. Place chicken breasts
in shallow pan and pour mixture over top. Marinate for 20-30
minutes. Preheat grill to medium-high. Place chicken on grill and
cook 6-7 minutes per side or until internal temperature reaches 165F.
Remove chicken from grill and let rest for 3 minutes before serving.
Serve with smashed yams, pg 123 and simple greens, pg 112.
Serves 4.

Chicken Breast Marsala

4 pieces chicken breast, boneless and skinless
¼ cup brown rice flour
2 tbsp grape seed oil
1 cup cremini mushrooms, sliced
2 cloves garlic, minced
½ cup Marsala wine
½ cup organic chicken stock, low sodium
1 tsp freshly cracked pepper
1 tsp sea salt

Preheat a non-stick pan to medium-high. Add grape seed oil. Place brown rice flour in bowl and carefully dredge chicken breasts in rice flour and place in pan. Cook until just brown, about 4-5 minutes. Turn chicken breast. Add garlic and mushrooms and cook for 4-5 minutes. Add wine and stock. Turn heat to low and simmer for about 5 minutes. Season with sea salt and freshly cracked pepper to taste. Serve with cauliflower mash, pg 114 and sautéed rainbow vegetables, pg 110. Serves 4.

Grilled Chicken Breast on Confetti Vegetables with Spicy Avocado Cream

4 pieces chicken breast, boneless and skinless
½ cup red pepper, diced
½ cup yellow pepper, diced
½ cup green onion, diced
½ cup carrots, diced
2 cups beluga black lentils, cooked
2 cloves garlic, minced
3 tbsp EVOO
Sea salt and freshly cracked pepper to taste
Spicy Avocado Cream, page 171

Preheat grill to medium-high. Rub chicken with 1 tablespoon of EVOO and season with sea salt and freshly cracked pepper. Place chicken on grill and cook 5-6 minutes per side or until internal temperature reaches 165F. Remove chicken from grill and keep warm. Heat a sauté pan to medium-high. Add EVOO, peppers, onions, carrots, lentils, and garlic. Cook the vegetables for about 5 minutes or until just tender. Keep warm. To serve, divide vegetables onto 4 warm plates covering bottom. Place chicken on top of vegetables and top with 1 tablespoon of spicy avocado cream sauce.

Chicken Breast with Artichokes and Wild Mushrooms

4 pieces chicken breast, boneless and skinless
¼ cup brown rice flour
1 can artichokes, quartered
1 cup wild mushrooms (cremini, shiitake, oyster, etc.), sliced
2 cloves garlic, minced
2 tbsp grape seed oil
1 tbsp fresh lemon juice
½ cup organic chicken stock, low sodium
1 tsp freshly cracked black pepper
1 tsp sea salt

Preheat a non-stick pan to medium-high. Add grape seed oil. Place brown rice flour in bowl and carefully dredge chicken breasts in rice flour and place in pan. Cook until just brown, about 4-5 minutes. Turn chicken breast and add artichokes, mushrooms, and garlic, cook for 4-5 minutes. Add stock and lemon juice. Turn heat to low and simmer for about 5 minutes. Season with sea salt and freshly cracked pepper to taste. Serve with smashed yams, pg 123. Serves 4.

Almond-Crusted Chicken Breast

4 pieces chicken breast, boneless and skinless
½ cup almond meal
1 egg, beaten
2 tsp Italian seasoning
1 tsp freshly cracked pepper
1 tsp sea salt
2 tsp coconut oil

Preheat oven to 350F. Use coconut oil to grease sheet pan. In a small bowl, combine all dry ingredients and mix well. Carefully dredge chicken breasts in egg and then into almond meal, coating evenly. Place chicken on sheet pan and place in oven. Bake until chicken is golden brown, about 30-40 minutes, or until internal temperature reaches 165F. Let rest 3-4 minutes and serve. Serve with smashed yams, pg 123 and asparagus with woodland mushrooms, pg 120. Serves 4.

Chicken and Cashew Stir Fry

1 lb chicken breast, boneless and skinless, cut into 1 inch cubes
1 cup sweet onion, diced
1 cup red sweet pepper, diced
1 cup carrots, diced
1 cup cashews
2 cups fresh spinach
2 tbsp coconut oil
1 tbsp lite teriyaki sauce
2 tbsp filtered water
2 cups brown basmati rice, cooked

Heat a non-stick skillet to medium-high. Add coconut oil to pan. When hot, add chicken. Cook chicken stirring frequently about 5 minutes. Add all vegetables to sauté pan and cook until vegetables are tender, about 5 minutes. Add spinach, teriyaki sauce, and water. Cook until spinach is just wilted. To serve, place ½ cup hot rice on 4 warm plates, then top with chicken and vegetables. Serves 4.

Oven-Roasted Rosemary Turkey Breast

3 lb turkey breast, boneless, skin on
2-3 cloves garlic, chopped finely
1 tbsp fresh rosemary, chopped fine
Sea salt and freshly cracked pepper

Heat oven to 400F. Rinse turkey and trim excess fat. Lift skin from turkey slightly and slide garlic and rosemary under skin. Season the outside of turkey with sea salt and freshly cracked pepper. Place in roasting pan and roast in oven for 20 minutes. Reduce heat to 350F and cook until internal temperature reaches 165F, about 45-55 minutes. Remove from oven and rest for 5 minutes. Use leftovers for lunches and salads. Serve with cauliflower mash, pg 114 and asparagus with scallions and woodland mushrooms, pg 120. Serves 4.

1 Pan Chicken with Peppers and Rice

4 chicken breast boneless, skinless, cut into 1 inch pieces
1 tbsp EVOO
1 red pepper, seeded, stem removed and cut into 1 inch pieces
1 yellow pepper, seeded, stem removed and cut into 1 inch pieces
1 can (26 oz) plum tomatoes
2-3 cups chicken stock, low sodium
1 cup brown basmati rice
2 tsp all purpose seasoning mix

Heat a large braising pan to medium high. Add EVOO. Season chicken with all purpose seasoning and add to pan with peppers. Cook for 4-5 minutes stirring often. Add plum tomatoes and chicken stock. Reduce heat and bring to a simmer. Add brown basmati rice. Simmer on low until rice is tender about 30- 40 minutes. If recipe becomes too thick add more chicken stock. Serves 4.

Grandma Rosie's Turkey Steak Burgers

1 lb all natural ground turkey breast
1 tbsp Dijon mustard
2 tbsp horseradish
1 egg, beaten
½ cup almond flour
1 tsp freshly cracked black pepper
1 tsp sea salt
1 tbso EVOO

Combine all ingredients in a large bowl and mix well. Season with sea salt and fresh cracked pepper. Divide turkey into four portions and press into patties. Place patties on film-lined plate and place in freezer for about 5-10 minutes. Preheat grill to medium-high. Rub turkey burgers with the EVOO. Place burgers on grill and cook until internal temperature reaches 165 degrees, about 4-5 minutes per side. Turkey burgers can also be prepared in a pan if you do not have a grill. Serve with sweet potato fries, pg 125 and flash fried French green beans, pg 119. Serves 4.

Zesty Oven Roasted Chicken

1 3 lb chicken, trimmed of excess fat
1 tsp all purpose seasoning
1 tsp cajun seasoning
1 tsp Italian seasoning

Pre heat oven to 425 degrees. In a small bowl, combine the spices. Remove any giblets from chicken and clean chicken of any excess fat. Place chicken in roasting pan and rub spice mixture onto the chicken. Place chicken in oven and roast for 15 minutes then reduce temperature to 350 degrees. Roast chicken for about 45 minutes or until internal temperature reaches 165 degrees. Remove from oven and let rest for 5 minutes. Serve with smashed yams, pg 123 and steamed broccoli. Serves 4.

Chicken and Shrimp Gumbo

3 tbsp EVOO
6 pieces chicken thighs, skinless, boneless
1 cup onion, diced
1 pablano pepper, seeded, diced
½ cup celery, diced
5 garlic cloves, diced
1 cup dry red wine
1 quart chicken stock, low sodium
2 cups water
2 tsp cayenne pepper
1 can tomatoes (28 oz), diced, drained
½ pound medium wild shrimp, peeled and deveined
1 tsp black pepper, ground
1 tsp sea salt
1 cup brown basmati rice

Heat a large pot to medium high. Add oil and chicken. Cook chicken for 5 minutes or until well browned. Flip chicken and cook for 3 minutes. Reduce heat to medium and add onion, celery, pepper and garlic. Cook for 5 minutes stirring frequently. Add wine, chicken stock, water, pepper and tomatoes and rice. Turn heat to medium low and simmer for 15-20 minutes. Add shrimp and simmer for about 15 minutes. Test rice to see if tender. If rice is still hard simmer a few more minutes until tender. If gumbo seems too thick add more water or chicken stock. Serves 4-6.

Beef

Grilled Balsamic Grass-Fed Sirloin Steak

4 pieces grass-fed sirloin steaks (4 oz each)
2 cloves garlic, minced
2 tbsp EVOO
1 tbsp balsamic vinegar
1 tsp freshly cracked black pepper
1 tsp sea salt

Combine all ingredients, mix well, and pour over steaks in shallow pan. Marinate for 20-30 minutes. Preheat grill to medium-high. Place steaks on grill and cook about 4 minutes per side or until internal temperature reaches 140 degrees (medium). Remove steaks from grill and let rest for 3-4 minutes before serving. Steaks can also be pan seared or oven roasted. Serve with sweet potato home fries, pg 124 and steamed fresh asparagus. Serves 4.

BBQ Beef Brisket

3 lb grass-fed beef brisket, trimmed of fat
2 cloves fresh garlic, minced
¼ cup sweet onion, minced
1 bottle chili sauce, low sugar
1 quart beef stock, low sodium
1 tsp freshly cracked pepper
1 tsp sea salt

Preheat oven to 350F. Place brisket in baking pan and top with garlic and onion. Add chili sauce and ½ of beef stock. Stock should be about 1 inch deep in pan, Season the beef with sea salt and freshly cracked pepper. Cover with foil and place in oven. Bake for 1 ½ hours, then remove from oven and carefully turn meat over in pan. Add additional stock if liquid is less than 1 inch deep in pan. Replace foil and place back in oven. Bake for an additional 1 ½ hours. Check beef for doneness after 1 additional hour. Beef brisket is done when fork inserts easily. Let rest for 5 minutes. Slice beef and serve with sauce. If sauce is too thick, thin with hot stock. Serve with flash fried green beans, pg 119 and sweet potato fries, pg 125. Serves 4-5.

Sunday Pot Roast

3 lb grass-fed beef chuck roast, about 1 ½ inches thick
1 cup baby carrots
1 cup celery, cut into 1-inch pieces
1 cup sweet onions cut into 1-inch pieces
1 cup button mushrooms
2 cups sweet potatoes, cut into 1-inch cubes
4 cloves fresh garlic, chopped
1 quart beef stock, low sodium
2 tsp freshly cracked pepper

Preheat oven to 350F. In a large shallow baking pan, place half the vegetables on bottom. Place beef on top of vegetables, then add remaining vegetables. Pour beef stock into pan and sprinkle the pepper over the beef. Cover dish with foil and place in oven. Bake for about 3 hours, checking often to make sure beef stock has not evaporated. If stock evaporates before beef is finished, just add more. Beef will be finished when fork inserts easily. Let rest for 5 minutes and serve. Serve with a mixed green salad, pg 68. Serves 4-5.

Portobello Mushroom Meatloaf

1 lb ground turkey
8 oz grass-fed lean ground beef
¼ cup sweet onion, diced
¼ cup celery, diced
½ cup Portobello mushrooms, diced, pan browned, and chilled
1 egg
½ cup almond meal
½ cup almond milk
1 tsp Italian seasoning
1 tsp sea salt
1 tsp black pepper
2 tbsp ketchup, low sugar
¼ cup quinoa, cooked

Preheat oven to 350F. Combine all ingredients except ketchup and quinoa. Mix well. Place meatloaf in baking pan and form into a 2 ½ inch deep rectangle. Place in oven and bake for 40 minutes. Remove from oven. Spread ketchup on top of meatloaf and sprinkle with the quinoa. Place back in oven and cook for about 15 minutes or until internal temperature reaches 165F. Remove and let rest for 5 minutes. Serve with roasted cauliflower, pg 113 and a mixed green salad, pg 68. Serves 4.

Beef and Broccoli with Pineapple Tamarind Sauce

1 lb grass-fed beef sirloin, cut into 3 inch by 1 inch strips
3 cups broccoli florets
1 tbsp coconut oil
¼ cup water
1 tbsp tamarind concentrate
1 cup beef stock, low sodium, warm
¼ cup red wine vinegar
½ cup golden pineapple, chopped fine
2 garlic cloves, minced
1 tbsp fresh ginger, grated

For the pineapple tamarind sauce, heat a saucepan to medium. Add the vinegar and pineapple and bring to a simmer. Cook until thickened like a syrup. Reduce the heat to low and stir in the pre-heated beef stock, then stir in the tamarind, garlic, and the ginger. Bring to a simmer and cook for 5 minutes. With a hand blender, blend sauce until smooth.

Heat a large sauté pan to medium high and add coconut oil. Add beef and cook for 5 minutes stirring frequently. Add broccoli and water and cover. Cook until water has evaporated about 4 minutes. Add the pineapple tamarind sauce and cook for a few minutes stirring often. Serve over ½ cup brown basmati rice. Serves 4.

Pork

Herb and Pecan Crusted Pork Tenderloin

1.5-2 lb piece pork tenderloin, trimmed of fat
1 tsp dried basil
1 tsp dried oregano
1 tsp dried rosemary
1 tsp dried thyme
¼ cup pecan meal
1 tsp freshly cracked pepper
1 tsp sea salt
1 tbsp whole grain mustard
1 egg

Preheat oven to 425F. In food processor, combine herbs and pecan meal. Blend well. Remove from processor and place in shallow container. Set aside. In small bowl, add mustard and egg and mix well. Coat the pork in mustard mixture and then coat heavily with pecan mixture. Place on baking sheet and bake in oven for 10 minutes at 425F, and then lower to 350F for 15 minutes. Remove the pork from oven when internal temperature reaches 145F. Let pork rest for 5 minutes, slice, and serve. Serve with roasted cauliflower, pg 113 and a mixed green salad, pg 68 with rainbow vegetables, pg 110. Serves 4.

Grilled Boneless Pork Chops with Creamy Mustard Sauce

2 pc boneless pork loin chops, (8 oz each)
1 tbsp EVOO
2 tsp Italian seasoning
2 tbsp mustard cream sauce pg 165

Pre heat outdoor grill to medium high. Place pork chops on a plate and rub with EVOO and Italian seasoning. Place on hot grill and cook for 4-5 minutes per side. Pork chops will be done when internal temperature reaches 145 degrees. Remove pork chops from grill cover with foil and let rest for 5 minutes. To serve, place 1 pork chop on a warm plate and top with 1 tablespoon of creamy mustard sauce. Serve with smashed yams, pg 123 and flash fried green beans, pg 119. Serves 2.

Slow Roasted Pulled Pork

2 lb piece pork sirloin
1 tsp garlic powder
1 tsp onion powder
1 tsp paprika
1 tsp sea salt
1 tsp black pepper
½ tsp cumin
BBQ sauce, pg 162

Preheat oven to 325F. Mix all dry ingredients together. Place pork in shallow baking dish. Rub dry ingredients all over pork, then add about ¾ inch of water to pan. Cover with foil and place in oven. Bake for 2 ½-3 hours, checking often to make sure water does not evaporate. Add more water if pan becomes dry. Pork will be done when fork pulls pork apart easily. Serve with 1 tablespoon BBQ sauce and sweet potato fries, pg 125 with beans and greens, pg 111. Serves 4.

Bacon-Wrapped Pork Tenderloin

1 pork tenderloin, trimmed of fat
4 slices bacon
1 clove garlic, peeled and cut in half
Sea salt and freshly cracked pepper

Preheat oven to 400 degrees. Rub garlic all over pork tenderloin.
Wrap pork tenderloin with bacon, making sure bacon overlaps.
Placed bacon-wrapped pork tenderloin on a baking pan with
overlapped part facing down. Season with a little sea salt and fresh
cracked pepper. Roast in oven until internal temperature reaches 145
degrees, about 30-40 minutes. Remove from oven and let rest for 5
minutes. Slice and serve with herb zucchini fries, pg 116, sautéed
rainbow vegetables, pg 110 and creamy horseradish sauce pg 156.
Serves 4.

Roast Pork Loin with Balsamic Beets and Pears

1-3 lb boneless pork loin
2 tsp all purpose seasoning
1 tbsp EVOO
2 cups red beets, peeled and cubed
1 cup pears, peeled, seeded and cubed
1 cup balsamic vinegar
1 tsp chili pepper flakes, optional

Heat oven to 400F. Trim pork loin of excess fat. Place pork loin in roasting pan and rub with EVOO and season with the all purpose seasoning. Place pork loin in oven for 20 minutes. Reduce heat to 350F and cook until internal temperature reaches 150F, about 35-45 minutes. Remove from oven, cover with foil and let rest for 5 minutes.

Place beets and balsamic vinegar in sauce pan. Bring to a boil and reduce heat to a simmer. Simmer beets for 5 minutes. Add pears and cook until vinegar is reduced to about a ¼ cup.

To serve, slice pork loin and place on warm plate. Top with the balsamic beets and pears. Serve with cauliflower cous cous, pg 115 and oven roasted rainbow vegetables, pg 110. Serves 4-6.

Vegetable Entrees

Zucchini Linguini with Grape Tomatoes, Italian beans and Spinach

3 large zucchini, spiralized
1 tbsp EVOO
2 cloves of garlic, minced
1 can cannellini beans
1 cup grape tomatoes
1 cup spinach
6-8 fresh basil leaves, chopped
1 tbsp grated parmesan cheese
Sea salt and fresh cracked black pepper

Cut the Zucchini with a spiralized cutter to look like linguini. Heat a medium size sauté pan to medium and add EVOO and garlic. Cook for 2-3 minutes. Add zucchini, beans and tomatoes. Cover and cook for 3-5 minutes. Add spinach and basil and cook until spinach is just wilted. Season with sea salt and fresh cracked pepper. To serve, divide zucchini linguini on to two warm plates and top with the parmesan cheese. Serves 2.

Polenta with Braised Baby Kale and Grilled Fresh Tomato Sauce

2 cups organic stone ground corn meal
½ tsp sea salt
1 tsp garlic powder
6-7 cups vegetable stock, low sodium
2 tbsp EVOO
2 cups baby kale, washed
½ cup water
1 tbsp grapeseed oil
1 cup grilled fresh tomato sauce, pg 166

In a medium pot add corn meal, sea salt, garlic and vegetable stock. Stir to remove lumps. Slowly bring to a simmer stirring often. Continue to stir and cook over medium low heat until broth is absorbed and corn meal is smooth, about 20 minutes. Add 1 tablespoons of EVOO to a 9 x13 baking dish and coat well. Pour polenta into the pan and allow to set or firm until cool, about 20 minutes. Once cooled, cut polenta into 12 squares.

Heat a sauté pan to medium high. Add 1 tbsp of grapeseed oil. Place 6 squares of polenta in pan and cook until crisp and light brown. Turn polenta and repeat. Remove polenta from pan and keep warm. Reduce heat to medium and add the baby kale and water. Cook until baby kale is wilted about 3-4 minutes. Season with a pinch of sea salt and fresh cracked pepper. To Serve, divide baby kale on to two warm plates. Place 3 slices of grilled polenta on top of baby kale. Pour 1/2 cup grilled fresh tomato sauce on top of polenta. Serves 2.

Spicy Cauliflower Chili Stuffed Peppers

1 (15 oz) cans great northern beans, rinsed and drained
2 cups cauliflower, chopped
½ cup celery, chopped
½ cup onions, chopped
4 cloves garlic, minced
½ cup corn
1 (4 oz) can roasted green chilies, drained, diced
2 tbsp red pepper sauce
1 tbsp EVOO
1 tbsp chili powder
1 quart vegetable stock, low sodium
Sea salt and freshly cracked pepper to taste
6 large peppers, tops cut off and seeded
6 tbsp plain Greek yogurt
¼ cup green onion, chopped

Heat a large stock pot to medium-high. Add the EVOO, cauliflower, celery, onions, garlic, and chilies and cook about 5 minutes. Add remaining ingredients (except greek yogurt and green onion) and simmer for 30 minutes, or until vegetables are tender. Carefully remove half of soup and blend in a food processor. Place pureed soup back into pot and simmer for 10 additional minutes. Season the chili with sea salt and freshly cracked pepper. Fill peppers with chili and place in a glass baking dish. Bake for 15 minutes at 350 degrees. Remove from oven and top each chili filled pepper with 1 tablespoon of plain Greek yogurt and chopped green onion. Serve with a mixed green salad, pg 68. Serves 6.

Black Bean and Sweet Corn Cakes with Roasted Red Pepper Cream

1 can black beans, drained
½ cup sweet corn
2 tbsp green onion, chopped
1 tsp cayenne pepper
1 egg
1 tbsp whole grain mustard
½ cup almond flour
2 tbsp grape seed oil

In a food processor add the black beans and corn. Pulse a few times. Add the black bean and corn mixture to a bowl and combine with the green onion, cayenne pepper, egg, mustard and almond meal. Mix well. Place in refrigerator for 30 minutes. To prepare, heat a medium size sauté pan to medium high and add the grape seed oil. With a 2 oz scooper, scoop black bean mixture into a ball and place in pan. Flatten gently with a spatula. Cook each side until golden brown about 4 minutes per side. Serve on a bed of simple greens, pg 112 and 1 tablespoon of roasted red pepper cream sauce, pg 168. Serving size is 2-3 cakes.

Sauces and Toppings

BBQ Sauce

12 oz can tomato sauce, no salt or sugar added
½ cup of water
½ cup balsamic vinegar
¼ cup worcestershire sauce
1 tbsp dijon mustard
2 tbsp coconut crystals
½ tsp onion powder
½ tsp garlic powder
½ tsp mustard powder
1 tbsp chili powder
¼ tsp cayenne pepper
½ tsp salt

Mix all ingredients together in small sauce pan. Bring to a boil, stirring frequently. Turn to low and let simmer for 10 minutes. Cool and refrigerate. Serving size is 1 tablespoon.

Cocktail Sauce

1 tbsp fresh all-natural horseradish
1 cup ketchup, low sugar
2 tsp fresh squeezed lemon juice
1 tsp hot sauce (optional)

Combine all ingredients in small bowl and mix well. Refrigerate for 15 minutes before serving. Serving size is 1 tablespoon.

Creamy Horseradish Sauce

1 cup plain Greek yogurt
1 tbsp horseradish
¼ tsp garlic powder
½ tsp sea salt
¼ tsp freshly cracked black pepper

In small bowl combine all ingredients and mix well. Serving size is 1 tablespoon.

Creamy Mustard Sauce

1 cup plain Greek yogurt
2 tsp Dijon or whole grain mustard
½ tsp garlic powder
½ tsp sea salt
¼ tsp freshly cracked black pepper

In small bowl combine all ingredients and mix well. Serving size is 1 tablespoon.

Grilled Fresh Tomato Sauce

4 large fresh tomatoes
1 tbsp grape seed oil
2 garlic cloves, peeled
4-6 leaves fresh basil
1 tbsp fresh parsley, chopped
1 tsp sea salt
1 tsp fine ground black pepper

Preheat outdoor grill to medium-high. Wash tomatoes and dry. Rub tomatoes and garlic with grape seed oil. Place tomatoes and garlic on hot grill and cook until dark brown. Tomatoes will look blistered and semi burnt. In a blender add tomatoes, garlic, salt, pepper, basil, and parsley. Blend on high until smooth. Remove sauce from blender and place in a sauce pot. Bring to a simmer and cook for 10-15 minutes or until desired thickness. Sauce can be frozen for later use. Serving size ½ cup.

Italian Meat Sauce

1 lb ground turkey breast
8 oz turkey Italian sausage
½ cup onion, chopped
2 cloves of garlic, minced
1 tsp Italian seasoning
1 can (26 oz) ground tomatoes
2 tbsp EVOO
1 cup water
1 tsp sea salt
1 tsp fresh cracked pepper

Heat a large sauce medium high. Add the EVOO, meat, onion and garlic and cook until brown. Add tomatoes, Italian seasoning, salt, pepper and water. Simmer for about 20-30 minutes. If sauce is too thick add more water. Serve with spiralized vegetables. Serving size ½ cup.

Roasted Red Pepper Cream

1 cup plain Greek yogurt
1 tbsp roasted red peppers
¼ tsp garlic powder
½ tsp sea salt
¼ tsp freshly cracked black pepper

Combine all ingredients into a tall mixing cup. Blend well with handheld blender. Serving size is 1 tablespoon.

Mango Salsa

1 cup mango, diced
¼ cup red pepper, diced
¼ cup red onion, diced
1 tbsp cilantro, chopped fine
1 tbsp jalapeno pepper, diced (warning, use rubber gloves during preparation)
1 tbsp lime juice
1 tbsp rice wine vinegar

Combine all ingredients in mixing bowl. Mix well. Refrigerate for 1 hour before using. Serving size 1-2 tablespoons.

Cucumber, Tomato, Red Onion and Pablano Salsa

½ cup English cucumber, diced
½ cup tomato, diced
¼ cup red onion, diced
1 tbsp pablano pepper, diced (warning, use rubber gloves during preparation)
1 tbsp balsamic vinegar
1 tsp fresh basil, chopped fine
½ tsp sea salt
¼ tsp ground white pepper

Combine all ingredients in mixing bowl. Mix well. Refrigerate for 1 hour before using. Serving size 1-2 tablespoons.

Spicy Avocado Cream

1 avocado, ripe, peeled, pitted and cut into ½ inch chunks
1 cup plain Greek yogurt
1 tbsp key lime juice
1 tbsp jalapeño pepper, diced (warning, use rubber gloves during preparation)
1 tsp cilantro, chopped fine
Sea salt and freshly cracked pepper to taste

Slice avocado in half and remove pit. Scoop out avocado meat from skin and place in food processor. Add yogurt, lime juice, jalapeño, cilantro, a pinch of sea salt and fresh cracked black pepper. Blend until smooth and creamy. If sauce is to thick add a little water.
Serving size 1 tablespoon

Mediterranean Olive Tapenade

2 cups mixed olives, pitted
1/3 cup roasted red peppers, chopped
1 tbsp sweet onion, chopped
1 garlic clove, chopped
1 tbsp fresh sweet basil, rough chopped
1 tbsp fresh parsley, rough chopped
2 tbsp extra virgin olive oil

Combine all ingredients in a food processor. Pulse until olive mixture is finely chopped. Season with fresh cracked pepper. Keep refrigerated. Serving size 1-2 tablespoons.

Tartar Sauce

1 cup Vegenaise® mayonnaise
1 tbsp fresh lemon juice
1 tbsp dill relish
½ tsp freshly cracked pepper

In small bowl combine all ingredients and mix well. Refrigerate for 15 minutes before serving. Serving size is 1 tablespoon.

Desserts

Note: For the desserts, only eat on occasion, like 1-2 times per week after you have lost your desired weight. Do not get into a habit of eating desserts every day.

Chocolate-Dipped Strawberries

1 pint strawberries, washed and dried
3 oz dark chocolate, 72% minimum
1 tbsp coconut oil

In a glass bowl add chocolate and coconut oil. Place in microwave and heat for 30 seconds. Stir. Repeat as necessary until chocolate is just melted and smooth. Be careful not to overheat as chocolate will get lumpy (curdle). Dip strawberries one at a time in chocolate and place on parchment paper lined plate. Refrigerate. Serving size is 3-4 strawberries.

Frozen ABC Bites (Almond Banana Chocolate)

2 bananas (more green than yellow) cut into ½ inch slices
¼ cup raw almonds
2 oz dark chocolate 72% minimum
2 tsp coconut oil

In a glass bowl add chocolate and coconut oil. Place in microwave and heat for 30 seconds. Stir. Repeat as necessary until chocolate is just melted and smooth. Be careful not to overheat as chocolate will get lumpy (curdle). Place sliced bananas on parchment paper-lined plate. Top each banana with one almond. With a spoon pour melted chocolate over almond and banana. Place in freezer for 1 hour. Serve frozen. Serving size is 3-4 bites.

Coconut Crunch Balls

3 oz dark chocolate, 72% minimum
2 tsp coconut oil
¼ cup raw walnuts, chopped
¼ cup shredded coconut, unsweetened

In a glass bowl add chocolate and coconut oil. Place in microwave and heat for 30 seconds. Stir. Repeat as necessary until chocolate is just melted and smooth. Be careful not to overheat as chocolate will get lumpy (curdle). Add walnuts and shredded coconut and mix well. Refrigerate until mixture is just firm, about 10 minutes. With a ½ oz scooper, scoop the chocolate mixture and form individual balls. If balls start to fall apart, form with your hands. Place balls on parchment paper-lined plate. Refrigerate for 1 hour. Serving size is 2 coconut crunch balls. Makes 6-8 balls.

Almond Coconut Crêpes with Raspberries and Cinnamon Maple Cream

1 cup Greek yogurt, plain
2 tbsp 100% maple syrup
½ tsp cinnamon
1 pint raspberries
¼ cup almond flour
¼ cup coconut flour
3 eggs
½ cup almond milk
¼ cup water
1 tbsp butter melted (grass-fed)
¼ tsp sea salt
Coconut oil

Mix yogurt, maple syrup, and cinnamon together and refrigerate.
Whisk together eggs. Add almond flour, coconut flour, milk, butter,
and sea salt. Mix well, making sure there are no lumps. Heat a 7-inch
non-stick pan to medium and brush with a little coconut oil. Pour ¼
cup of batter into the pan. Tilt or swirl the pan to evenly distribute
the batter, making a circle. Flip the crêpe when set and top is still
shiny, about 20-30 seconds. Cook for an additional 15 seconds.
Place crêpes on a plate and let cool. To serve, fill each crêpe with 2
tablespoons of raspberries and 1 tablespoon of maple cream. Roll
crêpe or fold over and drizzle with a little bit more maple cream. Top
with a few fresh raspberries and a sprinkle of cinnamon. Serving size
is one crêpe. Makes 5 crepes.

Acknowledgments

Thank you to my family;

My wife Michele who several times a week would ask "how is the book coming along or is the book done yet." She was also my recipe tester and would let me know if she did not like something.

My daughter Nicole who struggled with migraines and a dairy allergy. We worked together and simply changed her diet and pretty much eliminated these issues. She also helped test numerous recipes.

My son Johnny while at college put together the website www.rehealthyourself.com. I could not have done this without you. He has found an interest in food and is studying Food Science and Technology.

My sisters Jane and Julia for the first round of editing and trying recipes.

My sister Joann who kept encouraging me to share my recipes with others and who loves fresh fish and seafood.

My brother Jim who has always asked for new recipes and who loves cooking out on the grill.

Online Resources

1. Smoking. www.helpguide.org search smoking

2a. Sleep. www. Bettersleep.org
2b. How Sleep Loss Adds to Weight Gain.
http://well.blogs.nytimes.com/2013/08/06/how-sleep-loss-adds-to-weight-gain

3. Alcohol consumption. www.cdc.gov/alcohol

4. Stress. www.mayoclinic.org search stress management

5. Good Carbs vs. Bad Carbs. http://www.webmd.com/diet

6. Franken Wheat. http://www.huffingtonpost.com/dr-mark-hyman/wheat-gluten

7. Nuts for Weight Loss.
http://www.ncbi.nlm.nih.gov/pubmed/14574348

8. Green Tea: University of Maryland Medical Center
https://umm.edu/health/medical/altmed/herb/green-tea

9a. Food Labels: Institute of Food Technologists. http://www.am-fe.ift.org/cms
9.b FDA
http://www.fda.gov/Food/GuidanceRegulation/GuidanceDocuments
RegulatoryInformation/LabelingNutrition/ucm456090.htm

10. CSPI, http://www.cspinet.org/reports/chemcuisine.htm#letter-S
"chemical Cuisine"

11. CSPI, February 24, 2010. Salt-Water-Soaked Chicken Not at all Natural, Says CSPI

12. www.usda.gov/organic

13. Environmental Working Group. www.ewg.org

Quotes for Motivation

"The first and best victory is to conquer self"
Plato

"You must do the things you think you can not do"
Eleanor Roosevelt

"You may delay but time will not"
Ben Franklin

"Life itself is the proper binge"
Julia Child

"The food you eat in private shows up in public"
Anonymous

"The most difficult thing is the decision to act, the rest is merely tenacity"
Amelia Earhart

"The worst diet is the one that makes you fat"
Anonymous

"Your body is a temple not a drive thru"
Anonymous

"If food is your best friend it is also your best enemy"
Edward Jones

"Don't dig your grave with your own fork and knife"
English proverb

General Index

Recipe Index